THE PSYCHOSOCIAL EDUCATION OF NURSES:
THE INTERPERSONAL DIMENSION

For my children, Paul, Helen and Susan
and Sue, my adopted parent

The Psychosocial Education of Nurses: The interpersonal dimension

WITHDRAWAL

JOSIE GREGORY
BA (Hons), PhD, RGN, SCM, Dipl. Nurs., PGCEA, Dipl. Hum. Psycho.
Department of Educational Studies
(Human Potential Research Group)
University of Surrey
Guildford

Avebury

Aldershot · Brookfield USA · Hong Kong · Singapore · Sydney

Published by
Avebury
Ashgate Publishing Ltd
Gower House
Croft Road
Aldershot
Hants GU11 3HR
England

Ashgate Publishing Company
Old Post Road
Brookfield
Vermont 05036
USA

British Library Cataloguing in Publication Data

Gregory, Josephine
    The psychosocial education of nurses : the interpersonal
    dimension. - (Nursing)
    1 . Interpersonal relations 2 . Nursing - Psychological aspects
    3 . Nursing - Social aspects
    I . Title
    610 . 7 ' 301

    ISBN 1 85972 345 4

Library of Congress Catalog Card Number: 96-83712

Acknowledgement: Grateful thanks for permission to reproduce 'The Concept Indicator Model ' by Strauss, A., in *Qualitative Analysis for Social Scientists, 1987, p.25 Cambridge University Press.*

Printed and bound in Great Britain by Ipswich Book Co. Ltd., Ipswich, Suffolk

Contents

Figures   viii
Acknowledgements   x
Preface   xi

Part One: Introduction   1

Chapter 1   The history and context of this research   3
Personal biography   5
Reluctant learners   11
The development of the research questions   13
What is nursing?   14
Humanistic psychology and the education of adults   19
Humanistic psychology   19
Humanistic psychology and the caring relationship   22
The education of adults   25
The philosophy of the School of Nursing and
experiential education   28
Interpersonal skills training in nurse education   34

Chapter 2   Research philosophy and methodology   39
The choice of a constructivist paradigm   39
The constructivist paradigm   42
Applying the constructivist paradigm   43
The research methodology - grounded theory   46
The use of the literature in grounded theory   49
The stages of grounded theory   50
Methods used in grounded theory   56
Indepth intensive interviews   57
Observation in the natural setting   59

Chapter 3   Applying grounded theory   63
Selection of the research site   63
The ward working context   65
The educational working context   67
Formal access   68
Gaining access to participants   69
Sampling   70
Practical procedures surrounding intensive interviews   71
Initial sorting of data into codes and categories   75

Part Two: Discussion of findings   83

Chapter 4   The educational relationship   85
The core category: With-holding self as a strategy for self-management   87
'Living the contradiction' in education   88
Learning about self   94
Emotional education   94
'Belonging' in the learning set   104
Trusting self and others as an educative process   105
Mutual feedback   110
Peer group support   112
Disclosing self to others   119
The place of the psychological contract   127

Chapter 5   Interpersonal skills training   133
Interpersonal skills training in the School of Nursing   134
Self awareness and empathy   136
Communication skills as emotional contact   139
The therapeutic (enabling) relationship   142
Attitude development   145
Assertiveness training   146
Group learning of interpersonal skills   155
Interpersonal skills training in reality   163

Chapter 6   Interpersonal relationships amongst nurses on the wards   171
Conforming to try to belong to the ward team   172
Fast work is good work   174
Working as a team   182
The professional shield   201
Presenting a united front   201
Respecting authority and hierarchical control   208
Dimensions of the professional shield   211
Power and control   213

Dimensions of the professional shield   211
Power and control   213
Core categories and basic psycho-social processes   227

Chapter 7 Conclusion   233
Summary of the research   233
Revisiting core categories - The basic socio-psychological process   235
Consequences for the education of nurses   242
Consequences for nursing practice   246
A review of the methodology   249
Looking forward   253

Appendices   255
Appendix A The College curriculum: the interpersonal skills strand   257
Appendix B The analysis of data   259
Appendix C Structuring of time and interpersonal relationships   282

Bibliography   *285*

Figures

Figure 1.1   The proposed interpersonal skills strand   8
Figure 1.2   The phenomenological field of nursing   14
Figure 1.3   The "fenced-off" area of study   15

Figure 2.1   The Indicator-concept model   47

Figure 3.1   Ascriptive categories   76
Figure 3.2   Initial theoretical categories   78

Figure 4.1   Mapping the elements of the substantive theory of
              "With-holding self as a strategy for self-management"   86
Figure 4.2   With-holding self, as a strategy for
              self-management (1)   88
Figure 4.3   Patient-centred curriculum and student-centred
              educational processes   91
Figure 4.4   Internal variables linked with trust   109
Figure 4.5   External variables influencing trust   110
Figure 4.6   Co-variant factors influencing self-disclosure in groups   122
Figure 4.7   Factors influencing an "enabling" learning environment   125
Figure 4.8   The negative group learning environment   126
Figure 4.9   The psychological contract   129
Figure 4.10   With-holding self as a strategy for self-management (2)   130

Figure 5.1   A training skills model   149
Figure 5.2   Interrelationship between the interpersonal processes
              and the educational processes   163
Figure 5.3   The link between the psychological contract
              and interpersonal skills training   167
Figure 5.4   The parameters of "Respecting"   168

Figure 6.1	Category: Conforming to try to belong to the ward team	173
Figure 6.2	Theoretical coding on "Team work on the wards"	183
Figure 6.3	Tension between personal needs, environmental support and work ethos	187
Figure 6.4	Functional empowerment cycle	193
Figure 6.5	The dysfunctional (dis-empowerment) cycle	194
Figure 6.6	The dimensions of factors which create tension in conforming to try to belong to the ward team	200
Figure 6.7	Characteristics of the professional shield	211
Figure 6.8	The relationship between power, control and conflict	214
Figure 6.9	Mapping the elements of the substantive theory of "With-holding self as a strategy for self-management"	228
Figure 6.10	The negative feedback loop	229
Figure A-1	Indicators of the category: Facilitating personal learning	280

Acknowledgements

My appreciation and thanks to the many people who have supported my efforts during the five years of this study. In particular to Professor Judith Lathlean, Dr. Ricky Lucock, and Dr Paul Tosey for their encouragement, critical appraisal and moral support.

My thanks to my research support group, Dr Anne Lee and Dr Anne Riggs for their patience and guidance. My deep appreciation to the nurses, both tutors, staff nurses and to the student nurses who took part in this study: the gift you shared with me of your experiences relating at the interface between your inner world and your working world was essential for this study to succeed.

To Sue, and the family I shared under her guidance in the "Monday Group". Thank you Sue, and Janice, Shona, Caro, Jeanne, Pauline, Anne, Angie, Ann and Ali for your support, and Rose, for listening.

Thanks to my life long friends, Sharon and Alex Milne and family as well as Sister Kathryn Pinkman, for "staying separate" from this research. This enabled me to realise there was another important world of friends and family where I could for sacred hours be myself.

Most importantly to my children; Paul, Helen and Susan for their love, support and understanding.

Preface

This book is a report of a study which was initiated as a result of a concern that the philosophy and practice of facilitative interpersonal relating espoused in pre-registration nurse education was not transferring with ease into educational interactive teaching and learning processes nor to the practice of nursing, particularly between nurses themselves.

The research focused on:

a)   what constituted interpersonal relationships for the nurses studied,

b)   how the education of nurses addressed interpersonal relationships in teaching and nursing practice,

c)   how the development of interpersonal relationships as therapeutic enabling behaviour was practised among nurses themselves in educational and hospital ward practice.

A grounded theory approach (after Glaser and Strauss 1967) was used to discover what were the socio-psychological processes guiding how nurses related to each other.

A total of 176 nurses were sampled in this research. Thirty one nurses from student nurses to tutors in the a College of Nursing and trained nurses on some of the wards of a general hospital engaged in the study. This was followed by theoretical sampling with those same nurses and with other nurses outside the research site. The main method used was unstructured intensive interviews, many informal interviews, group discussions with some non-participant observations and use of curriculum documents.

The main findings were that nurses felt emotionally and behaviourally ill equipped to form enabling (socio-psychological) relationships with each other, and for the most part unwilling to be `enabling' to each other. In nurse education socio-psychological education in the form of Interpersonal skills training was given little priority over the 'clinical' curriculum and most tutors felt unable to teach the interpersonal curriculum experientially. Students recognised the need to develop interpersonal "enabling" skills; however, most did not demonstrate an investment in learning 'how to be enabling' in experiential education. The possible reasons for the lack of ability or lack of investment in developing "enabling" interpersonal relating were identified as core processes of personal vulnerability and fear of intimacy. These fears were shielded by the basic socio-psychological process of **With-holding self as a strategy for self-management** in which nurses seemed to be engaged. This was 'a holding back' from intimacy; that is being honest, spontaneous and creative as defined by Berne (1972) (Appendix C)

Aligned with the 'With-holding' and in some cases a manifestation of 'with-holding' was the other basic socio-psychological process identified, which was: the 'Professional shield' as a self-protective socio-psychological mechanism protecting against personal rejection, (real or imagined) and its auxiliary category: 'Conformity to try to belong to the ward team' as a strategy to counteract the perceived over-use of hierarchical power and control mainly within the ward team.

Fear of rejection and fear of intimacy were core categories which gave rise to the defensive strategies which nurses used in their interpersonal relationships with each other.

As a result of these findings, some more definite questions could be asked which would form the bases of further research. One question addressing the socio-psychological relationships among nurses could be: What is the investment for nurses (as a profession) in maintaining unsatisfactory interpersonal relations which maintain a state of dis-empowerment?

There is a recommendation for nurse educators generally to work within an educational psychological learning contract for interpersonal skills training, and that such training be called psychosocial education to give it more prominence and status in the curriculum.

Interpersonal relationships are influenced by the personal attributes which individuals bring to a relationship; their level of self-awareness, interpretative frames of reference, their values and attitudes, beliefs and constructs, their behaviour and skills as well as their energy and state of being (Mulligan 1993a: 8), hence the personal dimension will be a constant companion to the interpersonal dimension. This research sits within the discipline of social psychology as it is concerned with the behaviour of people in the presence of others in social situations.

The book is laid out in two parts. Part 1 includes Chapters 1 to 3 containing the research aims, the context in which the research was done, the research design, a map of the research process and initial analysis of data, while Part 2 is formed by Chapters 4 to 7 containing the theoretical analysis of the research data and a discussion on the findings.

In Chapter 1 the reasons why the interpersonal dimension between nurses was chosen as the area of study are discussed. In addition a broad canvas is painted covering the educational and nursing philosophy which were essential influencing factors in the research field during the active inquiry phase of the research. In Chapter 2 a rationale is offered for the choice of a constructivist research paradigm, and specifically why grounded theory was chosen to access the psychosocial dimensions of the interpersonal issues underpinning nurses' relationships with each other. Chapter 3 is primarily a descriptive account of how grounded theory was used in this research and the educational and ward context in which the study was done. In Chapter 4 a synthesis of the data on the interpersonal dimension between tutors and student nurses in the School of Nursing is offered with emphasis on the significant basic sociopsychological processes uncovered within their social relationships. The developing substantive theory around the personal and interpersonal relationships on general wards in one general hospital with the basic sociopsychological processes found form the substance of Chapter 6, together with integration of the theoretical categories discussed in Chapter 4. In Chapter 5 the research participants' perceptions of the interpersonal skills training are discussed with reference to the educational curriculum and how this linked to personal awareness and interpersonal skills behaviour as experienced by the research participants. The final chapter re-visits and discusses the theoretical categories forming the substantive theory found in this research. The social and psychological parameters of the interpersonal relationships amongst general nurses are reviewed and the implications of the findings are discussed. Recommendations for implementation of the research findings are offered with reflections on possible further lines of research.

Appendix B formed a complete chapter in the original research report and is offered here as an appendix for the interested researcher as examples of the microanalysis of verbatim data in grounded theory. The interview material is sorted into open codes, theoretical memos and then early theoretical categories for the purposes of generating a substantive theory.

PART ONE
Introduction

1 The history and context of this research

The basis of the practice of any service-oriented group lies in the beliefs and values that are held by that group. (Pearson & Vaughan, 1986, p.34)

Introduction

This chapter sets the scene for this research by opening up for scrutiny the many dimensions which impinge on the world of nursing both at a process level for nurses and within the structures and functions of nursing. A brief overview will be offered here of the different areas of concern with more detailed discussion occupying different sections of the chapter. One of the main concerns is the influence of humanistic psychology (discussed more fully later) within nurse education and practice. Rowan describes humanistic psychology as:

> ..a way of doing science which includes love, involvement and spontaneity. And the object of this science is not the prediction and control of people's behaviour, but the liberation of people from the bonds of neurotic control, whether this comes from outside (in the structures of our society) or from within. (Rowan, 1988, p. 3)

Rowan's definition of humanistic psychology includes 'a way of doing things' that indicates action processes and the quality of these processes. It also emphasizes an intention: 'the object is to... liberate' which is both directed internally (intrapersonal) and externally (interpersonal, social and cultural) in the process of liberating the individual, and the means of effecting such change is through an educational process of engaging with people in a facilitative manner rather than by imposition. These various emphases give a clear indication that humanistic psychology has a strong personal and interpersonal dimension, an educational focus and an end product of a caring liberating process for individuals.

Nursing as a quality of the interpersonal relationship between the nurse and patient gradually emerged from the above ideology of individualism and humanism (Maslow, 1972, Rogers, 1983, Rowan, 1988) popularised in the fifties and sixties and brought into nursing under the guise of holistic individualised care (Peplau, 1952, Reed & Proctor, 1993) and the theory of adult education (Heron, 1974, 1977b, Knowles, 1978, Jarvis, 1985). How this ideology influenced patient care and the education of nurses will be discussed under 'Humanistic psychology and the education of adults' section of this chapter. The humanistic approach stresses the personal and interpersonal development of individuals so that they might be more self determining and effective in relationships with others. How nurse educators in this study embraced these concepts and turned them into curriculum content and learning outcomes will be discussed in this chapter and in Chapter 5. The reason why the interpersonal relationship dimension was chosen will be addressed in various ways in this chapter, looking at relationships from the author's personal experience to the philosophy of the educational and working practices within nursing. The main aim in this Introduction is to establish that nursing is an interpersonal process as the whole study stands on this premise. The way I have chosen to do this is to put forward the research participants' own responses when I asked them what nursing meant to them (see Chapter 3) and to support this with the literature.

When asked the question: 'What does nursing mean to you?' all of the participants interviewed responded; 'Nursing is about the quality of the interpersonal relationship between the nurse and the patient'. This interpersonal relationship was seen to have social, psychological, and behavioural dimensions within the continuum of health and illness. How nurses were prepared or prepared themselves for such relationships is one of the themes of this research. The central theme however, is how nurses related to each other.

This book will not report on studies of the direct nursing care of patients, yet without that focus there would be no reason for nurses to be trained and working together on the wards. As the role relationship between the nurse and the patient is constantly touched on, a definition of nursing will be offered under the section 'What is nursing?'. Nursing as professional practice will be included where appropriate.

The intriguing problems which led to this research will be described next to lead the reader into the context of the research in order to better understand the nature of the research inquiry.

4

Personal biography

This research had its genesis in personal teaching experiences which occurred over the three years following a teacher training course. This experience led to a concern for the appropriateness of creating learning experiences for nurses which were intended to be educative but which were not often perceived as educative by the participants.[1]

The following is a sequential summary of the three years experience. The 'new' Registered General Nursing course started with twelve weeks in the School of Nursing. The students spent most of that time learning about health and human relations which included personal and interpersonal development for themselves.[2]Experiential groupwork was used to teach self-awareness, communication skills and other relationship skills as part of the personal and interpersonal skills strand of the curriculum. (see Appendix A)

Visual observations of the group of students showed that they seemed very uncomfortable with the process of 'getting to know each other' using experiential exercises called ice breakers (Brandes & Phillips, 1978). They also expressed a dislike for the exercises developed for them to learn basic communication, assertion and empathy skills. They were agitated about the requirement for them to negotiate the educational content they needed to learn and the teaching methods employed; learning contracts, experiential learning, sharing project work, seminars and other forms of interactive teaching methods. This agitation was inferred by their silence or moans amongst themselves and the written comments in their evaluation forms. The students stated that they preferred to be lectured to rather than to interact with each other in the classroom and in effect, they preferred to keep their learning to themselves.

Drawing together my own and other tutor's observations and studying the feedback from the evaluation forms, the conclusion was that the students' 'resistance' to interacting and sharing their learning seemed to stem from:

a   Lack of structure of the introductory course.
b   Reluctance to participate in groupwork exercises.
c   The tutor's style of teaching personal development training, and
        inexperience in creating a supportive environment for learning.

Assumptions about students' ability and willingness to learn from one another in the classroom seemed unfounded. Small cohorts were friendly enough, but the dynamic of the large group (18 students) seemed hard to understand and manage.

My colleague and I worked hard with the group. It was an experiment both for us and for the students. The students did not appreciate being 'guinea pigs' either for the new curriculum or for the 'new' teaching methods and let this be known in indirect ways. By the end of the twelve weeks the students seemed more accepting of both the tutors and the experience. However this was more to do with moving on to studying clinical nursing which they perceived to be more relevant than the study of cultural, social and psychological aspects of healthy individuals. In the introductory block my colleague and I had tried to establish a more open and less hierarchical relationship with the students, role-modelling the belief that the education of adults can only be done between adults, where 'power' as parental power was at a minimum. The students did not seem to appreciate this form of equal and open communication style and could not relate to us in any manner other than hierarchical and what I later identified as 'distancing'. One of the reasons why they may have maintained this stance throughout the first year of their training was possibly a result of their experiences on the wards. Many of the students had difficulty practising their new found interpersonal skills with staff on the wards. They tried to influence decisions by negotiating their learning needs in the form of learning contracts, and their social needs in the form of off-duty requests. They also asked for rationale for nursing care and treatment, giving their opinion and their agreements and disagreements in a manner they perceived to be assertive. They learned that the ward culture seemed to encourage silent acquiescence, which in Fielding and Llewelyn's (1987) view, is detrimental to communication skills. In the hierarchical environment of the wards such a belief in interpersonal parity seemed foreign, so if the nurses spoke out they were labelled trouble-makers. Many of these students had a difficult time on their first wards, and they were extremely angry with the tutors for teaching them ideas and behaviour which 'got them into trouble'.

It was my contact with these angry and hurt students which initiated the concern about whether the educational content in the interpersonal skills strand as well as the experiential teaching methods were really what student nurses needed to work effectively on the wards. I was also concerned that the ward staff seemed to have different criteria for how students learned different types of skills. Developing clinical skills was expected and some mistakes were tolerated as part of the learning process, yet, learning and practicing interpersonal skills was not tolerated well and mistakes unacceptable despite the literature expounding on the need for good interpersonal skills. For me the issues of concern were:

♦ What might be going on in the learning group that creates uncertainty about group interactive skills learning?

♦ Were the students too inexperienced, (although some had come from other professions, such as social work and teaching, or previous adult work) to take part in the interpersonal skills training and interactive learning we were encouraging?

6

♦ Was the timing of the interpersonal skills training at a suitable juncture in the curriculum?

Although I had been teaching in nurse education for some years, teaching students as a tutor was a new experience, so it was difficult for me to separate out what was the normal pattern of student behaviour with their tutors and what was different about this group's way of working and relating with us and the new curriculum.

I was allocated to co-ordinate and to teach the next introductory course and from my experience of the previous group, I was as tentative and sensitive in teaching as the students' knowledge and experience would allow. There was still reluctance by both students and other tutors to engage in teaching techniques which encouraged students and teachers to reflect on their learning, and make that learning explicit by sharing it in the learning group. This introductory course was more structured than the previous one so there was less need for students to negotiate the course content which seemed easier for them to manage. Yet, it was still an upward struggle encouraging students to interact with each other in an enabling way. I intuitively felt the students' 'un-explained discomfort' (Sullivan, 1948) which is the unique characteristic of anxiety and found it difficult to engage them in participatory learning. At that time I was also involved in teaching more senior students 'management skills'. Their feedback as to their reluctance to engage in co-operative interactive learning was not dissimilar to the junior students. Many complained that they had a taste of self-awareness training and interpersonal skills in the introductory weeks of the course, with tutors using what they (the students) saw as superficial social skills training techniques which had little bearing on 'real' situations on the ward. They then did not re-visit the subject of interpersonal skills until the final management block of the three year course. The management block, however, clashed with their final written examinations and they were more concerned with preparation for passing the examinations than with focusing on personal and interpersonal changes. It seemed that when the interpersonal skills content was taught in the early stages of the course, the students would evaluate it as being ineffective as they did not have enough nursing experience to relate it to, but when it was done near the end of the course, they said it was too late to be of benefit and their examinations were more important. On the surface there was a great deal of logic to the students' arguments. However, the end result was the ineffectual implementation of the interpersonal skills strand and poor execution of curriculum aims with respect to the psychosocial development of the student within the educational context.

I pondered on this seemingly difficult problem for some months, then taking ideas derived from Kagan, et. al., (1986) and the NHS (National Health Service) Distance Learning Resource Unit (Townsend, 1983b, Marson, 1985, I decided to develop a sketch of key concepts (Figure 1.1) that could form a programme of interpersonal skills training which would thread in a spiral fashion throughout the curriculum (Bruner, 1960). The proposal was that the interpersonal skills strand would cover the subjects necessary and Marson and Townsend's (1983b) list of subjects would offer conceptual maps or models which would give theoretical and practical structure to the interpersonal skills strand. These conceptual models included Transactional Analysis, Gestalt, Neurolinguistics Programming, Co-counselling, Psychodrama and other personal and interpersonal relationship models. The sketch shown below in Figure 1. 1, was circulated to teaching colleagues for comments.

Figure 1. 1 The proposed interpersonal skills strand

The concept of self:	The socialisation process, (personal self awareness, person perception, body image, self esteem, personal needs and self-actualisation.
The self and others	Social perception, the social interpersonal context: roles, rules, values, norms, rituals and culture. Socialisation; the societal perspective; Verbal and non-verbal behavioural communication. Development of students in professional practice.
The social (professional) context:	Social network.Problem-solving. Counselling. Loss and adaptation. Assertiveness.
The organisational context:	Group dynamics, leadership styles, crisis intervention. The reality of change. Goal directed behaviour. Systems theory.

The concept of self....to move through above cycle again at a deeper level of inquiry as part of continuing professional training.

Teaching colleagues seemed unaware of most of the models in the proposal. Their responses to the proposals were supportive of my intentions, but very negative about the proposed programme itself. The main concern was that the theoretical models introduced seemed too specialised and therefore not suitable for general student nurses. As the models were new to the tutors, I could

8

understand how they assessed them as being too specialised. Another comment was that the proposed programme 'was a three year course in its own right' (according to one tutor) and 'there would not be enough time in the curriculum to devote to them' (according to another tutor), so that time seemed to be a concern as well as specialism of content. The rejection of the proposal was not a serious blow, other than a frustrated acceptance that 'the world will not change in a day' and a continuing reflection on 'is this what student nurses need or want anyway?' These first tentative questions planted the seed of this research: they are important questions which need answers.

Over the following 18 months teaching student nurses, one of the conclusion I drew was that students were not in a strong position to change the culture on the wards as they were the most junior people, with even less power to influence ward policy, custom and practice than auxiliary nurses. This was demonstrated very vividly in Melia's work on the socialisation of students into the profession (Melia, 1987, p.108). It seemed to me to be un-ethical to educate solely from below, intentionally or un-intentionally asking the students to become change agents when they had the least power to do so. This was a dilemma they had no right to have placed on them as they were too in-experienced to make informed choices about initiating second order changes, that is, influencing the system of nursing itself. The literature shows that student nurses soon reconcile this dilemma by siding with the staff on the ward (Melia, 1987) and using the college staff as scapegoats to justify their allegiance to service staff's needs.

I reflected that the best people to educate into interpersonal ways of being enabling on the ward were the trained staff. The hope was that if the trained staff were trained in interpersonal relationship skill and learned the value system of humanism, then by example, and active teaching, they could teach the students these same skills, or at the very least they would understand from their own educational experience what the tutors were aiming to do when teaching interpersonal skills as part of nursing principles in the new curriculum. Part of the value system of humanism can be summed up with Peplau's assertion that:

> It is likely that the nursing process is educative and therapeutic when nurse and patient can come to know and to respect each other, as persons who are alike, and yet, different, as persons who share in the solution of problems. (Peplau, 1988, p.9)

These principles were based on a participant relationship between nurse and patient, where the agenda is for the nurse to do nursing care with the patient, not to him or her. Teaching these principles to senior nurses which they could apply to junior nurses as well as to patients seemed to me to be the way to create both a therapeutic environment for patients and an educative environment for all nurses on the wards.

With my goal for effecting change in interpersonal relating now focused on the trained nurses I moved to a teaching post in the Department of Continuing (Nurse) Education. I took on particular responsibility for teaching the English National Board 998 course: Teaching and Assessing in Clinical Practice (1988) to senior clinical nurses, as well as coordinating and teaching other professional development courses to trained nurses in the health district.

During the next eighteen months, I ran many short courses on clinical and professional development for staff nurses, ward managers and other senior nurses. Many concerns touched on the interpersonal issues raised by students in basic nursing education and my main observation was that the power to change peer relationships in the ward, and to create a positive learning environment for student nurses was perceived by trained nurses, not to be within the power of the students but firmly in the hands of the ward managers and the long stay trained staff, yet they themselves felt that the power to change ward practice was dependent on those above them. This observation supported those of Fretwell (1982), Ogier (1982), Lathlean & Farnish (1984) and others and also links with Menzies' (1960, p.19) 'delegation of responsibilities up the managerial hierarchy'.

Many of the trained staff on the short courses I facilitated did seem to appreciate the interactive, experiential nature of our learning together once they became accustomed to it. They would say that it was a pity that student nurses coming on their wards did not seem to know how to articulate their learning needs or to be able to act with self-direction and confidence (in andragogical terms). However, the most challenging aspect of teaching the professional development courses which were more psychosocial than clinically orientated was facilitating the trained staff to articulate their own learning needs, create learning contracts and take part in experiential learning as part of interpersonal skills training. Yet these nurses would be expected to facilitate such learning with the students on the wards. It seemed a circular argument and I felt that I was going back to the original problem again. The phrase:

> If only we had been taught these interpersonal skills in this manner (interactively) when we were students it would have made life on the ward much easier to cope with. I would have felt more confident about how I related to staff and patients, (Ward Sister)

was one side of the coin, the other being:

> What is the point in us learning these things when we can't put them into practice, as we are too junior, it's the trained staff you have to teach. (Student)

At this stage I thought, `If I'm not careful, I could give up trying to make sense of the paradoxes which seem to be part of the fabric of nurses as a social or professional group.' Instead I chose to investigate the phenomenon further. Both senior nurses on the clinical services side and in the S.O.N.(1) had created the curriculum as part of a Joint Course Management Board, yet those who were being asked to practise therapeutic interpersonal relating had some difficulty in understanding and learning what those concepts meant and what skills they needed to put such concepts into practice.

My personal biography ends here with the completion of 18 months teaching in Continuing Professional Education. This was really a spiral of inquiry as it led me through cycles of experience at pre-registration to post-registration level in how nurses in one particular district viewed their interpersonal relationship skills and how they learned them or not.

Reluctant learners

The question stayed with me as to why students found intrapersonal and interpersonal development and practice difficult within the teaching and work environment. As a tutor in Continuing Education I learnt that the issues of interpersonal relationships seemed important to trained staff, yet they did not see themselves as being the main role models in competent interpersonal relating with each other or with students. By `reluctant learners' I came to include trained nursing staff in my workshops as well as students in their initial training.

The need to develop interpersonal therapeutic skills as part of giving good nursing care seemed to be accepted at an abstract level, however, how to develop such skills seemed problematic for all staff; tutors, trained nurses and students. I felt it to be important to investigate what was happening at a sociopsychological level of functioning among nurses that was influencing their interpersonal relationships. I was intuitively sensing a problem, so went out to look for one. (Lofland & Lofland, 1984, p.8) The classic work done by Menzies in 1960 on `The Functioning of Social Systems as a Defence against Anxiety' seemed to be manifested in terms of some of the avoidance strategies I was observing. Menzies, however, was addressing the relationship between the nurse and the patient and how nurses as a social system had created structures and functions as a defence against the anxiety inherent (according to Menzies) in the nurse / patient relationship. At a surface level those social systems had changed in the way nurses organised their work. This change included

11

allocating nurses to look after a specific group of patients for the whole of their shift and even for two or three days to build up relationships with patients rather than task allocation according to nurses' skills and seniority. Was this newer way of working and learning less anxiety provoking for nurses than in the years leading up to Menzies' study? If not, where was the anxiety being displaced or how was it being managed?

The tendency to link my observations to Menzies' work was attractive. It would have been convenient to find this as a possible solution, however, my preference was to explore what might be going on for people, rather than try to fit my tentative hypothesis into a ready made theory. In the process of selecting an appropriate methodology to explore what were the underlying sociopsychological issues between nurses I decided to go into the research field, holding back any biased views or 'bracketing'. (Spinelli, 1989, p.17. See Chapter 2) It felt important to find out how the people in the field, the tutors, student nurses and trained nursing staff perceived the issues of interpersonal relating amongst themselves and how the interpersonal skills training influenced how they managed their interpersonal relationships. As Kagan states:

> ...to do their job, nurses bring the interpersonal skills that work for them in their every day lives and apply them at work. But something happens when they do this. .....research into the effectiveness of nurses' communication and interpersonal skills have shown them to be sadly lacking. Even taking into account that hospitals (and other health care settings) are strange and unique places where strange things happen to people, it seems that nurses readily succumb to external and internal pressures to discard or distort their interpersonal skills. (Kagan et al., 1986, p.2)

Kagan gave no reason why nurses might discard or distort their interpersonal skills, rather she used the phenomenon to argue for the need to teach interpersonal skills in Colleges of Nursing. It would be interesting to explore aspects of the social settings as perceived by students, trained staff nurses and tutors which might account for the 'de-skilling' which was observed. To do this effectively the research needed to be exploratory, so a search for the appropriate research paradigm began and the method chosen is the subject of Chapter 2. For now, an indication of the research questions (or research focus) will be explored.

The development of the research questions

As stated earlier, this research arose as the result of difficulties I experienced in teaching interpersonal skills to nurses. As a nurse teacher trying to create a learning environment where students could learn about self awareness and interpersonal skills according to the curriculum, I encountered a 'tension' which seemed like resistance to the educative process. What puzzled me can be summed up thus:

a   What right had I, as a teacher to facilitate self-awareness and interpersonal skills training if both colleagues and many of the students did not seem to want them?

b   How did the students 'apparent difficulties' or 'reluctance' (my label) fit with the notion of willing participation (Heron, 1989a) and negotiated learning (Heron, 1977b, Knowles, 1978) espoused by humanistic educators and practitioners (Rowan, 1988 and others), and acknowledged by the School in their curriculum document? (School of Nursing (S.O.N. (1) 1986. p.82)

c   The course curriculum stated that self awareness and interpersonal skills were a necessary part of preparing nurses for their caring role, but did the student nurses and trained nurses see them as necessary and relevant?

d   If the self awareness and interpersonal skills content as stated in the curriculum were not relevant, what type (content) of personal and interpersonal skills development would nurses want, if any?

The questions rather tormented me as I perceived an ethical dilemma in continuing to teach curricular subjects without a firm commitment from both colleagues and students that such subjects were meeting the needs of individuals. I turned my puzzlement into two broad questions for this research:

1   What are your interpersonal relationships like, with each other as students, with tutors, with ward staff, with the patients?

2   Personal and interpersonal skills training is part of nurse education. How might such training raise personal and interpersonal relationship issues for you, both in the School of Nursing and on the wards?

These questions are more a "fencing-off" of the area of study (Stern, 1985, p.153) (Figures 1.2 and 1.3) rather than a more structured format of questions generally posed in social science research. Defining the area rather than pin pointing the questions is recommended in grounded theory as a way of `avoiding incorrect research aims', or `premature closure'.(ibid.,)

The discussion so far has opened up the curricular intention which was that nurses were expected to train in interpersonal skills to develop therapeutic relationships with patients (curriculum document S.O.N.(1) 1989). This intention, however, needs to be supported with more extensive discussion through different perspectives, such as the definition of nursing as well as exploring the underlying philosophy within the educational and practice setting. These will form the substance of the following two sections.

What is nursing?

Defining nursing with a simple sentence is difficult due to its multi-dimensional aspects embracing theories from many disciplines, practice in many contexts and relationships between those that nurse, those who are nursed and other health care professionals. These multiple dimensions are more easily seen diagrammatically as in figure 1. 2

Figure 1. 2 The phenomenological field of nursing

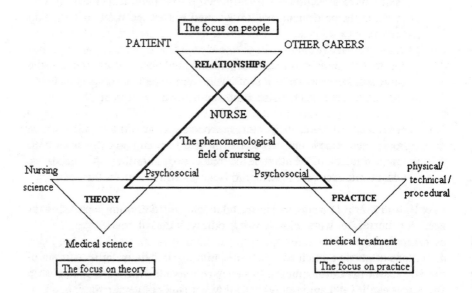

N.B. The "fenced-off" area of study (Stern, 1985) focusing on the psychosocial aspects of interpersonal relationships between nurses is more clearly seen in Figure 1. 3.

Figure 1. 3 The 'fenced-off' area of study

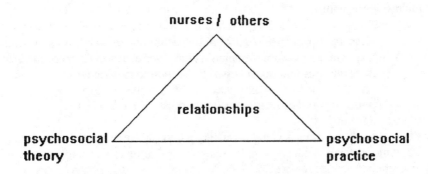

However, the relationship between nurses only exists as part of a greater relationship which is that between the nurse and the patient. A definition of that relationship is offered below:

> The unique function of the nurse is to assist the individual, sick or well, in the performance of those activities contributing to health or its recovery (or to peaceful death) that he would perform unaided had he the necessary strength, will or knowledge, and to do this in such a way as to help him gain his independence as rapidly as possible. This aspect of her work, this part of her function, she initiates and controls; of this she is master. In addition she helps the patient to carry out the therapeutic plan as initiated by the physician. She also, as a member of a medical team, helps other members, as they in turn help her, to plan and carry out the total programme whether it is for the improvement of health, or the recovery from illness or support in death. (Henderson in Harmer & Henderson, 1955, p.4)

As Hall (1982, p.1) states in his introduction, this definition 'speaks of the need for nurses to work closely with others'... and it recognises the key psychological role of the nurse for both patient and colleague. There are many definitions of nursing, often based on the philosophical stance of the definer as can be seen in the development of models of nursing. (King 1971, Roy 1976 and Roper et al., 1980 amongst others) However all would agree that nursing is about working with people, in an interpersonal way, (Travelbee, 1971, Alexander, 1983, and Skevington, 1984), that nursing is about caring, certainly physical caring which Roach (1984, p.42) emphasises must be combined with

15

the "personal, humanistic, spiritual motivation of caring that is the very basis of nursing". Roach goes on to say that, `caring is experienced transpersonally, that is, in relation to others in the environment.' Peplau's (1952) values preceded Roach's and were very similar, though Peplau brought a strong psychotherapeutic model to nursing and her definition fits her own philosophical stance:

> Nursing is a process, first of all. By this we mean that its serial and goal directed nature demands certain steps, actions, operations, or performances that occur between the individual who does the nursing and the person who is nursed....it is an interpersonal investigative, nurturing, and growth-provoking process. (Peplau, 1988, p.5)

And in the curriculum documents of the School of Nursing where this study was done is stated:

> Nursing is a dynamic process which embodies preventative, therapeutic and rehabilitative care of the individuals within the hospital and community irrespective of race, colour, class, creed or personal values. (S.O.N. (2) 1989, p.1)

The above definitions illustrate that nursing as an activity is mainly an interactive, interpersonal human process. Nursing has both qualitative and quantitative dimensions, the qualitative dimension including valuing of the person and the emotional quality of caring. (Llewelyn, 1984, Smith, 1992) The quantitative dimension includes physical care or tasks over time, technological care and material resources, where the focus of care is on treatment boundaries and cure (Hoy et al., 1986, p.42) as medically defined (see Figure 1. 2). Many theoretical models of nursing developed over the last 40 plus years incorporate issues of belief about human nature; about what nursing knowledge is; and the theory of nursing methods or approaches, for example, Peplau, 1952, King, 1971, Roy, 1976, Orem, 1980, and Roper et al., 1980. It is not the intention to extend the exploration of the definition of nursing in this section, but rather to concentrate more on the philosophical basis of nursing in a following section. What is important for this study is that if nursing is accepted as a psychosocial (Minardi & Riley, 1988) and therapeutic process and given equal importance to clinical caring, (Faulkner, 1980) (see Figure 1. 2, main inner triangle), then, for nurse tutors, the study of nurses' perceptions, knowledge and skills in these areas is a necessary pre-requisite to teaching interpersonal relationship skills to nurses.

To explore the concept of relationships I have chosen Laing's (1965) work and to a degree Buber's (1937) as opposed to others (Argyle, 1969 for example) as they are more congruent with the type of humanistic relationships defined by

Rogers (1967) and Egan (1982) appropriate to this study. Laing (1965), an existential phenomenologist and humanist, saw relationships as a person-to-person process where viewing the other as a person implies a different perspective on the part of the observer to viewing the other as a biological or mechanical entity. As he says:

> Now, if you are sitting opposite me, I can see you as another person like myself, without you changing or doing anything differently, I can see you as a complex physical-chemical system perhaps with its own idiosyncrasies but chemical none the less for that; seen in this way you are no longer a person but an organism (Laing, 1965, p.21).

Here Laing is proposing that we have a choice about how we view others, either as objects or people. To see the other as 'another human being' is to attribute to her/him the same inner world we hold for ourselves. We acknowledge that 'the other person' will hold personal values, beliefs and feelings which are idiosyncratic and of significance to him/her which manifests in their behaviour. It means to attribute to the other person experiences which form his/her unique reality, or way of perceiving their world, and respect how the person makes sense of that, rather than to treat the other(s) as objects upon which we can enforce interpretations.

As nurses claim to hold the same phenomenological humanistic stance derived from a Laingian philosophy, then to be congruent, they would need to incorporate this perspective in their relationships with patients. Carl Rogers, who was of the same psychological persuasion as Laing, said:

> To withhold one's self as a person and to deal with the other as an object does not have a high probability of being helpful. It is the way that the attitude is perceived by the client that is crucial. (Rogers, 1967, p.41)

Clay (1986) gave a succinct historical account of the different philosophical persuasions under which nursing has operated over the past 150 years. Using Bevis' (1982) identification of the four major philosophical systems; from asceticism, to romanticism, pragmatism, and in this era, humanism with existentialist roots, Clay argues that traces of all the philosophies can be found now within the nursing profession. An existential humanistic perspective has dominated Western nursing theory and to a lesser extent practice since the early eighties. This is reflected in the theories of Rogers (1967), Egan (1982) and Heron (1990) emphasizing a 'helping relationship' and in the sentiments nurses are encouraged to bring to relationships from The Royal College of Nursing's 'Position Statement on Nursing: In Pursuit of Excellence,' (1987, pp.8-9). The commissioning team identified three main principles which they

17

offered as core concepts on which the nurse-patient relationship is based; equity, respect for the person, and caring which they explained as:

Equity:
> about power and political relationships, which needs skills in negotiating and influencing, self-awareness, assertiveness. Knowledge of role identification and interpretation of roles.

Respect for the person:
> Stems from a value system which prizes others simply because they are human beings.

Caring:
> This is shown through human warmth, patience, gentleness, compassion, companionship, and through the nurse's ability to build a relationship, and a level of communication which is personal to the individual and his family in an atmosphere which enables sensitive private issues to be discussed.

These principles emphasise the interpersonal nature of nursing rather than in more objective organismic or functional terms'. (Skevington, 1984, p.30) The principles are useful as they describe some of the interpersonal behaviours as well as internal processes in the form of sentiments which individuals need to bring to their nursing. Further, the RCN position statement encourages nurses to have a political awareness not just in their relationships with patients, but within the wider occupational and social arena. I believe the above RCN statement sits comfortably with Rogers' (1967) definition of an enabling relationship; of positive regard, empathy, and respect. These sentiments were also highlighted by Graham (1983), James (1989) and Smith (1992) as emotional involvement versus social distance in which caring is seen as emotional labour. The notion of equity is similar to Heron's (1989a) three political modes in facilitative practice; hierarchy, co-operation and autonomy, that is; the power the helper has over the client, the power shared by helper and client, and the autonomous power within the client. Heron maintains that all three forms of power need each other in a balancing way as appropriate for a healthy dynamic to be sustained between helper and client. (adapted from Heron, 1989a, pp.6-7) This section on defining nursing has of necessity included humanistic concepts which reflect the cultural influence of person-centredness of our time. The following section develops this approach in more detail, specifically linking it with the education of adults where nurse education is placed.

Humanistic psychology and the education of adults

In this section some of the fundamental beliefs of humanism will be discussed, then links will be made with the theory of the education of adults and nurse education in particular.

The link between humanistic psychology (which will be defined in the next section)) and adult education was firmly forged by Rogers (1972) who viewed adult learning as personalised learning, that is, involving all the internal capacities of the individual in the learning experience, emotional, cognitive, intuitive and sensing faculties as well as behaviour. The value which Rogers placed on learning was heavily influenced by his own humanistic perspective. Butterworth's (1984, p.55) list of principles which he adapted from humanistic psychology and which he suggested would form a humanistic approach to nursing education, reflects Rogers' (1972) stance. These humanistic principles are that nurse education:

*   should be student-centred rather than patient treatment focused,
*   should facilitate personal growth through humanistic methods,
*   should examine characteristics of a helping relationship,
*   should be a shared learning experience.

The above axioms are held as non-negotiable principles by the purists within humanistic education and will be developed further on. The complexity of holding a particular strong stance, whether it is pragmatism or rationalism, dualism or holism, lies in the need to be conscious of the philosophical premises on which the person's belief stands. That is, that the philosophical beliefs span belief about human life and how it is valued; about the nature of knowledge; about the nature of learning and about the nature of relationships. Therefore the educational ontology, epistemology, methodology and processes in nurse education need to be internally homogeneous within a same belief and value system as much as they are externally heterogeneous with other value systems and approaches. By virtue of making the above statement explicit I am also demonstrating the believe that there are multiple perspectives with different value systems and approaches. The importance of a relativist ontology (Guba & Lincoln, 1989, p.84) will emerge again in Chapter 2, but for now the emphasis is that the humanistic approach values the richness of multiple worldviews as shall be discussed more fully in the next section.

Humanistic psychology

Humanistic psychology was born out of a reaction to behaviourism and psychoanalysis, as the former was seen as mechanistic and empty of inner personal experience, while the latter was seen to hold a pessimistic outlook on human nature (Arac, 1988). Humanistic psychology on the other hand focuses on personal change as an educative liberating process, rather than control or repression of people's thinking, feelings and behaviour.

While nursing is often described as holistic, meaning an integration of the whole person, mind, body and spirit, (which is given due attention in practice), it says nothing about the manner in which nursing is done, that is, the personal qualities and beliefs with which the nurse views and cares for a patient or client holistically. Holism is important as a social construct to counter-balance the Cartesian splitting of body from mind and soul. (Pearson & Vaughan, 1986, p.35) I would argue, however, that holism without humanistic values would not qualify as a `caring perspective' for nursing; it would seem like a body without a soul, or labour without love. (James 1986, Smith, 1992) When viewed in this light of a caring respectful attitude, humanism brings a moral dimension to relationships. (Learn, 1990) Buber (1937), developing the I-thou dialogue in interpersonal relations, built his existential stance on mutual respect, dignity and appreciation of the rich uniqueness of individuals. (Learn, 1990, p.236) The development of the Buberian qualities described above, seems a moral obligation for those in professional therapeutic relationships as such is the inherent nature of therapeutic relationships which I see supported in the RCN (1987) position statement.

These Buberian qualities are embedded in the beliefs underpinning humanistic psychology, which are that all individuals have an inherent ability to develop all aspects of their personality: personal, interpersonal and transpersonal. The motivation to develop into self-directing autonomous people, interdependent with others, is seen as a liberating force:

> Growth takes place when the next step forward is subjectively more delightful, more joyous, more intrinsically satisfying than the previous gratification with which we have become familiar and even bored; that the only way we can ever know what is really right for us is that it feels better subjectively than any alternative. The new experience validates **itself** rather than by any outside criterion. (Maslow, 1972, p.43)

So personal development is seen as a necessary ingredient to the I-thou facilitative relationship important in a humanistic philosophy of nursing education and practice and needs to form part of the theoretical foundations of nursing studies. Individuals and individual needs are the important pivot points on which the humanistic approach is based. This individualism is founded on an existential philosophy where the `key concern for investigation is the existence as experienced by man as an individual. (Misiak & Sexton, 1973, p.71)

20

It is important to stress the origins of humanistic psychology as it allows for a more comprehensive appreciation of how the humanistic principles and methods can be used both educationally, therapeutically and socially. Maslow (1970, p.52), (often quoted as the Father of Humanistic Psychology) described a theory of motivation based on individual needs. He argued that the individual strives to get all needs met, from physical needs of sleep, physical activity, sexual activity, food and so on, to emotional support and security, and beyond that to a sense of his /her own destiny (autonomy) and self-sufficiency, to creative expansion into transpersonal (cosmic) and spiritual awareness. Maslow's needs hierarchy gives the impression of lower order needs followed by higher order needs with the lower order needs, that is, physiological needs needing to be satisfied before the individual aspires to higher order (social and aesthetic) needs. While this is likely developmentally, the adult can move through any of the needs intentionally and in that sense is empowered to address needs as appropriate rather than impulsively or instinctively (that is, out of conscious control).

However humanistic psychology is not just an individualistic approach as is sometimes imagined. It has a distinctive social awareness, honouring both individual differences as well as cultivating collective harmonious living and responsibility for environmental issues. The principles, derived from existentialism, are co-operation, humility and responsibility and are not to be confused with more recent 1970s "pop psychology and self-grandiosity". (Spinelli, 1989, p160) Having said that, "existentialism is concerned with human longing and search for meaning within the self." (Learn, 1990, p.237) Therefore an existentially based education encourages self-discovery as a way of developing this distinctive individual and social awareness and behaviour.

The shades of difference between humanistic psychology and its existential phenomenological roots over the past 30 years is that the former has developed a more optimistic view of human nature than the latter as well described by Deurzen-Smith when she wrote:

> The humanistic psychology's assumption that human beings are `basically positive creatures who develop constructively, given the right conditions,' is to be decried, rather, `the existential attitude is that people may evolve in any direction, good or bad, and that only reflection on what constitutes good or bad makes it possible to exercise one's choice in the matter. (Deurzen-Smith, 1988, pp.56-57)

Evidence of a political and organisational move towards individualism which in its conceptual form seemed humanistic in nature was found in the production of hospital mission statements introduced in the early 1980s. This in turn was supported by hospital managers and nurse educators encouraging ward nursing staff to devise ward philosophies which were patient-centred with a humanistic stance, such as:

1   adults are autonomous, independent and responsible for their own
         health...

2   people have the capacity to heal themselves, but may not have the
         knowledge to do so or be prepared to accept the responsibility. It is
         important to every individual to know how they perceive their own
         health.. or illness,.. in order to participate fully in their care. (S.O.N
         (1) ward philosophy, 1986)

Such statements support the rights of individuals to have their personal, social
and political needs and values taken into account as part of their total patient
care. This is a philosophy which is intended to empower the individual
receiving care as well as those giving care. Some would say that humanistic
ideas were hijacked by the politicians of the day who turned person-oriented
approaches into a consumer centred ideology which was put into action
through the White Paper 'Working for Patients' (HMSO, 1989). A glimpse into
the political backdrop in existence during this study seems important but will
be resisted because the emphasis in this thesis needs to stay with nurses and
how they relate to each other as they provide holistic care.

Humanistic psychology and the caring relationship

Carl Rogers (1951) spoke of the 'caring relationship' from a humanistic stance
when speaking of therapeutic encounters. He started from the viewpoint that
'In a general way, therapy (*meaning psychotherapy*) is a learning process' (op
cit., p.132) and in a later publication, goes on to say:

         The therapeutic relationship is only a special instance of interpersonal
         relations in general, and the same lawfulness governs all such
         relationships. (Rogers, 1967, p.39)

By lawfulness he appears to mean the same intentions and qualities the
individuals bring to the relationship whether it is therapeutic or educational.
There will be some change in emphasis between the helping relationship of
nurse with patient and teacher with students, yet again Rogers believed the
intentions and values to be the same in both relationships, as in helping
relationships generally, which are:

         That at least one of the parties has the intent of promoting the growth,
         development, maturity, improved functioning, improved coping of life
         of the other... (*further on*) a helping relationship might be defined as
         one in which one of the participants, intends that there should come

22

about, in one or both parties, more appreciation of, more expression of, more functional use of the latent inner resources of the individual. (Rogers, 1967, pp.39-40)

Part of Rogers' theory of personality and behaviour was derived from his own studies of adults in therapy. It was from the anti-psychiatric movement (Laing, 1965) of the 1950s and 1960s that humanistic ideas and practices gradually filtered through to psychiatric nursing in the 1980s where they were 'legitimised' by the General Nursing Council (then the statutory educational body for nurse education in England and Wales) when they endorsed the 1982 Registered Mental Nurse syllabus recommending humanistic principles and methods, both therapeutic and educational. In that syllabus, they also introduced the notion of the use of the self as a therapeutic agent as an essential concept in nursing. (Burnard, 1991, p.16) The General Nurse training syllabus gradually converted to humanistic principles, both in clinical nursing and general nurse education with the support of the validating bodies (the four National Boards for England, Wales, Scotland and Northern Ireland) under the new statutory structure of the United Kingdom Central Council for Nurses, Midwives and Health Visitors, (UKCC) which had taken over from the General Nursing Council in 1983. As Burnard (1991, p.17) reflected many of the leaders in nurse education of that time had been strongly influenced by the teaching and research of the Human Potential Research Group at the University of Surrey (then called the Human Potential Research Project), a centre for humanistic education and this influence was reflected in the curricular guidelines emerging from firstly the GNC followed by the ENB throughout the 1980s. As Koldjeski summarised:

> Professional nursing caring has to be embedded in a professional socialization process that emphasises both humanistic and scientific aspects of the therapeutic use of the self. (Koldjeski, 1990, p.48)

Such acceptance of humanistic values and methods into education was not unique to nurses, as Rogers' (1967) influence from psychotherapy into adult education generally spread from the USA to England by Rogers' own studies and with the work of Knowles (1978) and Heron (1977a). This can be seen with Rogers' definition of educational relationships and how it matches the definition of humanistic caring (Rogers, 1967, pp.39-40) According to Rogers:

> Attitudes of helper which is growth-facilitating will be acceptance - democratic with an ability to develop a person-to-person relationship; ability to understand the person's meanings and feelings (or an attitude of a desire to understand) **(empathy)**; a sensitivity to the person's attitudes; a warm interest without any emotional over-

23

involvement, **(positive regard)**. Trustworthiness is important if the relationship is to be helpful... which is about being congruent or transparent, that the helped person can see who you are as well as what you do, ie, **genuineness or congruence.** (ibid., 1967, pp.41-47)

From Rogers' definition above about the nature of [3]enabling relationships, I would conclude that the relationship is helpful if the intention is to improve personal functioning and / or growth and if the attitude and behaviour match that intention. What is being addressed here are the processes (both therapeutic and educative) with which the tutors and students perceive they are enacting the qualities of valuing the person and the person's learning needs. According to Hockey (1980, cit Alexander, 1983, p.31) 'the challenge for nurse teachers was the necessity that they educate for care', and she listed amongst qualities of caring; empathy and respect for individuals.

As can be seen, Rogers' definition of caring is invested in the personal qualities of the carer, particularly the psychotherapeutic carer. Rogers, who was influenced by Dewey's (1916) progressive education thought that some teachers would not have the promotion of (psychological) growth as their educational aim, yet the philosophy of the S.O.N.(1) of the research site, does state that personal growth is a positive attribute for the [4]therapeutic relationship nurses are asked to have with their patients. Rogers' (1983) views on education developed contemporaneously with those of Knowles, (1972) and Freire (1972), and were linked with Dewey's (1916 and 1938) progressive educational philosophy. Rogers advocated a move from traditional educational methods, particularly with professional education, to focusing on learning:

> We are, in my view, faced with an entirely new situation in education where the goal of education, if we are to survive, is the facilitation of change and learning. The only man who is educated is the man who has learnt to learn: the man who has learned how to adapt and change, the man who has realised that no knowledge is secure, that only the process of seeking knowledge gives a basis for security. Changingness, a reliance on process rather than upon static knowledge, is the only thing that makes any sense as a goal for education. (Rogers, 1983, p.120)

This facilitation of learning has been the challenge of adult education for the past thirty years and philosophically has been the main change in nurse educational thinking and direction over the same period of time. (Jarvis, 1986, Burnard, 1991)

The education of adults

The modern philosophical base which gave rise to humanistic educational thinking during the 1950s and 1960s has its origin in John Dewey's (1938) progressive education. The link between Dewey's educational philosophy with humanistic psychology and the education of adults can be traced to Dewey's commitment to valuing the individual's personal involvement in experiential learning. Dewey advocated a more proactive interactive learning approach in education between the learner and the teaching resources (of which the teacher is part, but only a part) which was grounded in the personal experience of the learner; `We shape all knowledge by the way we know it.. (subjectively)' and:

> I take it that the fundamental unit of the newer philosophy is found in the idea that there is an intimate and necessary relation between the processes of actual experience and education. If this is true, then a positive and constructive development of its own basic idea depends upon having a correct idea of experience. (Dewey, 1938, p.20)

Dewey (1938), Rogers (1967), Heron (1977c) and Knowles (1978) have pioneered approaches to the education of adults which are similar, in that they take account of individual life experience, the relevance of the educational content, and the method of teaching and learning. The theory of `how adults (best) learn' was named `andragogy' by Knowles (1978, pp.18-51) after he discovered the term used by European adult educators and philosophers in the 1950s. A debate about the difference between the education of children (pedagogy) and the education of adults (andragogy) as methodologies is not intended here. Jarvis (1986) critiques this at some length, and I agree with his argument that age related educational structures and approaches have more to do with historical and political influences than education per se. Jarvis goes on to say that education is a human process which needs to take account of principles which can be recognised as humanistic, and in this he is in accord with Rogers and Heron. Jarvis believes that:

> Education is about the art and science of helping humans learn. However there are differences in education when the philosophy of the person is analyzed. Nursing does require practitioners who are independent, self-directed persons, so that an understanding of the relationship between the philosophy of the person and the design of the curriculum in nurse education is important. (Jarvis, 1986, p.465)

Traditional education often termed `education from above' is seen as more politically/ socially controlling of learners and inhibitive to individual creativity (Dewey, 1938) whereas progressive education is seen as the `education of equals', (Knowles, 1978). In fact Durkheim's (1972) definition of traditional education emphasises the sociological perspective:

> Education is the influence exercised by adult generations on those that are not yet ready for social life. Its object is to stimulate and develop in the child a certain number of physical, intellectual and moral states which are demanded of him by the political society as a whole, and by the particular milieu for which he is specifically destined. (cit, Williamson, 1979, p.4)

Jarvis also looked at education from a sociological perspective, linking this with curricular models to illustrate the main differences between the two educations more easily. There he speaks of the two educations, that is the education of equals and education from above as having distinctly different aims, objectives, teaching methodology and assessment strategies. (Jarvis 1985) As Jarvis says in the same debate; education cannot be neutral, it is either the education from above, or the education of equals. He sees a tension between the aims of pedagogy which is about the `moulding' of the child to adopt societal norms and andragogy as an educational process whereby the personal development of the individual is the primary aim. He goes on to say;

> In nurse (professional) education there is a conflict of interest between the education of the person in the College of Nursing and the training for the job in hospital wards. (Jarvis 1985, p.45)

Combining the two educations is not considered a conflict of interest in nurse curriculum documents and yet was recognised as such by Dewey when he said:

> Mankind likes to think in extreme opposites. It is given to formulate it's beliefs in terms of Either-Ors between which it recognises no intermediate possibilities. When forced to recognise that the extremes cannot be acted upon, it is still inclined to hold that they are all right in theory but when it comes to practice matters circumstances compel us to compromise. Educational philosophy is no exception. This Either-Or is the opposition between traditional education and progressive education. (Dewey, 1938, p.17)

It seems appropriate to list some of the important assumptions which Knowles considered to be necessary for the education of equals as these complement Jarvis' stated above. Knowles asserts that the education of equals is based on the following premises:

Changes in self-concept:
> As the individual moves from dependency to increased independence (in learning). As the person voluntarily moves, in terms of self-

concept, from dependency, he becomes psychologically adult. He then no longer wants to be controlled by others and displaces this in resentment and resistance.

The role of experience:

As the individual matures he accumulates an expanding reservoir of experiences that causes him to become an increasingly rich learning resource, and at the same time provides him with a broadening base to which to relate new experiences. To a child, experience is something that happens to him, to an adult his experience is who he is. So in any situation in which that experience is being devalued or ignored, this is not just a rejection of the experience, but of the person himself.

Readiness to learn:

Adults are more ready to learn. It is not the case of learning what they 'ought to learn' as with children, but what they think they need to learn as relevant to their life, career and so on. The critical implication of this assumption is the importance of timing learning experiences to coincide with the learners' developmental tasks.

Orientation to learning:

adults tend to have a problem-centred orientation to learning. The reason for this is the timing of the learning to relevant here and now application.

(Adapted from Knowles, 1978, pp.58-59)

The ultimate motivation for adults is the need to maintain and develop their own self-esteem, which is the valuing of self, and which comes about when:

* the individual is able to define his own goals,
* the goals are related to his central needs or values,
* the individual is able to define the path to those goals. (Paton et al., 1985, p.63)

The above assumptions have considerable importance for adult educators and have formed the bases of many adult liberal educational programmes as well as Continuing Professional Development short courses (Gregory, 1993). How this is manifested in the School of Nursing (1) is best seen through its educational philosophy which will be discussed in the following section.

The philosophy of the School of Nursing and experiential education

The School of Nursing S.O.N.(1) where this research took place, held a philosophy which embraced humanistic principles and practices which are akin to Knowles' (1978) theory of how adults best learn. The philosophy of adult education links with experiential education in the minds of adult educators particularly through the influence of Dewey (1938), Lewin (1951) and Piaget (1971). Traditions of experiential learning trace their roots back to innovators of modern educational philosophy (Dewey, 1938), social and technological research (Lewin, 1951) and developmental cognitive psychology and learning theory. (Piaget, 1971) The internal homogeneity between progressive education, humanistic education, and experiential learning lies in the belief of the active learner, as one who has personal agency, in that he or she is self-directing, intrinsically curious and motivated to learn. The concept of personal agency is derived in this sense from Harré (1983) who states that being an agent means to conceive oneself as a being in possession of an ultimate power of decision and action. In educational terms the notion of personal agency can be best illustrated by Heron's definition of the educated person:

> ..an educated person is someone who is self-directing: that is, ..one who determines and is internally committed to what he conceives to be worthwhile objectives, to acceptable means of achieving them, and to appropriate standards of performance in achieving the objects by those means. Secondly, he is someone who is self-monitoring: he evaluates his own performance in the light of the standards he has set and becomes aware of the extent to which that performance fulfils, exceeds or falls short of those standards. Thirdly, he is someone who is self-correcting: he modifies his own performance, his standards, and means, or his objectives as experience and reflection appear to his considered judgement to require. (Heron, 1974, p1)

The professionally educated person would have the above capacity to self-assess, self-monitor and self-correct as a self-directed process which is part of being able to learn from and through experiences and knowing the skills of learning to learn. Such attributes are the hallmark of the educated person and are the focus of the education of adults.

Experiential education embraces the four functions of thinking, feeling, intuition and sensing which humans have of being in contact with the world. (Jung, 1977) Whereas Jung's four modes of being are limited in their explanation, Heron builds on them by postulating more comprehensively four modes of functioning;

- Affective-embracing feelings and emotions

28

- Imaginal-comprising intuition and imagery
- Conceptual-including reflection and discrimination, and
- Practical-involving intention and action. (Heron, 1992, pp.14-15)

These four modes are placed here to illustrate the holistic nature of humanistic learning theory which can be applied to learning processes whether in a therapeutic, educational or social and health care setting. Experiential education, Dewey's 'educative experiences', (1938, p28) implies engaging all modes of functioning if learning is to be an integrative experience for the individual. How these attributes are embraced within one nurse educational establishment can be seen in the School of Nursing's (S.O.N. (1)) philosophical statement and curricular intentions (1989) for the Registered General Nursing (RGN) course, under the heading of course structure where it stated that:

> It embraced the concept of valuing the uniqueness of the individual, and related nursing as a humanistic activity.

The curriculum document opened with a statement which mirrors andragogical thinking:

> Nurse education was a joint enterprise between the educationalists, and the clinical staff, and aimed to promote in the student, critical thinking, adaptability, responsibility and autonomy. (S.O.N. 1989, p.80)

Just at the time when this study started, the above philosophy was combined with the philosophy of another School of Nursing (S.O.N.(2), as the two amalgamated to form one College of Nursing (C.O.N. (1)). The addition included:

> The total learning experience gained by the student following this curriculum will enable her to become a Registered Nurse who is a competent and knowledgeable practitioner, capable of working autonomously and in collaboration with other professionals, with the capacity for personal growth and continued professional development. The philosophy is on student centred learning.

Here the College of Nursing explicitly speaks of personal growth and student centred learning, after Rogers (1951, Ch.4) and Knowles (1978) indicating that they are a necessary component of preparing to be a registered nurse. The curriculum document developed this theme further:

The Educational Unit believes that learning is a successful and enjoyable experience when learners are motivated and given freedom to question, negotiate learning methods, actively contribute to self and peer group learning and experiment within a psychologically safe environment. (S.O.N. (2) 1989, p.6)

However the tension between education from above and the education of equals was again highlighted:

The eclectic curriculum model has been selected with the central aim of providing a balance between too much emphasis on the `product end' or the opposite picture of the emphasis on `the process of learning' which sets no parameters upon the outcome of instruction. (ibid., 1989, p.81)

And in the same document:

Whilst respecting the above (teachers' professional autonomy in teaching style...) consideration is also directed to the ethos of a particular course. Thus teachers involved in courses where all the students are adults will need to be familiar with the rationale and skills required for facilitating learning within a framework of andragogy. (S.O.N (2) 1989, p.82)

The School of Nursing where this research was conducted is not unique in this philosophical stance, but rather is one example of how nurse education in general adopted a humanistic and andragogical philosophy of education (Clay, 1986). Another College of Nursing I worked in during this research, based its courses on the same educational philosophy of the empowerment of students which was reflected in curriculum documents, for example:

The learner is recognised as an adult with individual worthwhile knowledge, experience, skills, values, beliefs and needs. Participation of the learner in all stages of the learning process is fundamental. (College of Nursing (2) 1989, p.81)

and further on:

The values placed on andragogy will be confirmed by introducing students to the rationale and skills involved in assuming personal responsibility for achieving their learning objectives in the foundation unit. (ibid., 1989, p.82)

30

However the School of Nursing used in this research foresaw some resistance from students moving from a (possible) history of pedagogical education to an andragogical one when it stated in the curriculum document:

> It is recognised that this will not be a responsibility welcomed by the students in the early part of the course. Nevertheless this approach *(andragogical)* to learning is considered necessary and appropriate in order to achieve the intended course outcomes. (S.O.N.(2) 1989, p83)

The experiential approach to education described by Kolb (1984) is committed to empirical and experimental ways of teaching and learning. Experience is given a very high profile with encouragement to experiment with teaching nursing knowledge using innovative teaching methods within an andragogical framework. However, there is a need to explore what `experience' is, and how best to use experiences educatively. Dewey sounded a caution on this when he states:

> The belief that all genuine education comes about through experience does not mean that all experiences are genuinely or equally educative. Experience and education cannot be directly equated with each other. For some experiences are mis-educative. Any experience is mis-educative that has the effect of arresting or distorting the growth of further experience. An experience may be such as to engender callousness; it may produce lack of sensitivity and of responsiveness. Then the possibility of having richer experiences in the future are restricted. (Dewey, 1938, pp.25-26)

Dewey goes on to talk of experiences which have so little purposive structure that the disconnectedness one from the other dissipates the person's energy for learning and they become scatter-brained, no matter that the experiences may be temporarily enjoyable. The message is to create experiences of the right kind. In andragogical terms, this means offering experiences which will encourage learning to learn in a holistic fashion.

Educators in the School of Nursing in this study had the intention of offering `educative experiences' (S.O.N-1989, p.82) by advocating[5] participative teaching / learning methods as well as encouraging individual self-directed study and tutor/ peer groupwork, particularly for interpersonal skills training. The reason for their choice of experiential methods could be summed up in Heron's description of group experiential learning;

> ..an experiential group is one in which learning takes place through an active and aware involvement of the whole person, as a spiritual,

thinking, feeling, choosing, energetically and physically embodied being. (Heron, 1989a, p.11)

and experiential learning;

> Experiential knowledge is knowledge gained through action and practice. This kind of learning is by encounter, by direct acquaintance, by entering into some state of being. It is manifest through the process of being there, face-to-face, with the person, at the event, in the experience. This is the feeling, resonance level of learning (ibid., 1989a, p.13)

Certainly if experiential learning as described by Heron is to be holistic then it needs to move through the face-to-face encounter to the other levels mentioned earlier; the imaginal, conceptual and practical. The importance of learning and experience is evidenced by Kolb's offer of a working definition of learning:

> Learning is the process whereby knowledge is created through the transformation of experience. (Kolb, 1984, p.38)

This experience needs to involve learners opening their feelings, emotions, intellect, intuitive sense, and spiritual awareness to maximise the learning. Group learning would be the involvement of others in that process, with the sharing of responsibility for creating the experience, the sharing of learning and direct feedback to each other. This learning would span the concrete experience, reflection and critical reflection. Interpersonal skills training particularly lends itself to this type of educational process and will be discussed in a later section of this chapter. A major pathway to the exploration of feelings, emotions, intellect, intuitive sense and spiritual awareness is through emotional education. Heron separates feelings from emotions, seeing emotions as:

> ..the intense, localised effect that arises from the fulfilment or the frustration of individual needs and interests. This is the domain of joy, love, surprise, satisfaction, zest, fear, grief, anger and so on. Thus defined emotion is an index of motivational states. (Heron, 1992, p.16)

Ellis, (1973) believes that emotions are met and un-met beliefs and expectations. I offer these definitions of emotion to illustrate the complexity of emotions and because experiential learning is often referred to as emotional education or education of the affect (Heron, 1982). Feelings are seen by Heron (1992, p.16) as being transpersonal, that enable the person to connect at a sensory, and psychic level of awareness and which produce empathy, presence, resonance and so on. However he also agrees with others that feelings are sensory from the nervous system; like feeling hungry, feeling pain and so on (Heron, 1992). MacMurray (1935) considered the ideal action to be 'the spontaneous expression of feelings' *(emotions)* and goes on to say:

> The emotional life is not simply a part or an aspect of human life..it is the core and essence of human life. The intellect arises out of it, is rooted in it, draws its nourishment and sustenance from it, and is the subordinate partner in the human economy. This is because the intellect is essentially instrumental (MacMurray, 1935, cit Dunlop, 1984, pp.22-23).

As can be seen, emotions spring out of somatic experiences and according to Dunlop (1984, p.2) are better analysed phenomenologically rather than conceptually, that is, analysing the language or concepts of emotions.
Heron's definition of 'emotional competence' is when:

> a person [who] has it to be able to manage their emotions awarely in terms of the basic skills of control, expression, catharsis and transmutation...

He goes on to say:

> In every day living, emotional competence means being able to spot the stimulation of old emotional pain and to interrupt its displacement into distorted behaviour. So old hurt-laden agendas are not projected, nor transferred, into current situations. It means being able to spot institutionalised and professional forms of displacement, and to find ways of replacing them with more rational, flexible and adaptive behaviour. (Heron, 1992, pp.131-134)

Emotional competence is a crucial dimension in personal and interpersonal development for professional practice and will be referred to when discussing the interpersonal skills strand in nurse education. In this study participants used feelings and emotions synonymously; therefore the context will decide whether feelings as somatic experiences or emotions are being referred to.
This brief discussion on experiential learning helps to place it in the context of the andragogical philosophy with its associated humanistic values professed by the School of Nursing in this study. It is not intended to be comprehensive in terms of the practice of educational experiential learning. Apart from highlighting the origins and history, it seems more useful to find out how such principles were applied in practice in the School of Nursing. I want to conclude

this section with Rogers' definition of experiential learning with the underlying assumptions, as the elements he speaks of are fundamental principles informing this study. These are:

- ♦   It has the quality of personal involvement
- ♦   It is self-initiated (which is different from self-directed)
- ♦   It is (primarily) evaluated by the learner
- ♦   Its essence is meaning

(Rogers, 1972, p.276)

The assumptions underlying experiential learning which Roger identified were:

- ♦   Human beings have a natural potentiality for learning,
- ♦   Significant learning takes place when the subject matter is perceived by the student to having relevance for his own purposes,
- ♦   Much significant learning is acquired through doing,
- ♦   Learning is facilitated when the student participates responsibly in the learning process,
- ♦   Self-initiated learning, involving the whole person of the learner, feelings as well as intellect, is the most pervasive and lasting,
- ♦   Creativity in learning is best facilitated when self-criticism and self-evaluation are primary, and evaluation by others is of secondary importance,
- ♦   The most socially useful learning in the modern world is the learning of the process of learning, a continuing openness to experience, an incorporation into oneself of the process of change. (op. cit., pp.278-279).

How these principles were understood and applied in the School of Nursing particularly within the interpersonal skills training strand will be covered in the following section and in the discussions of findings in Chapters 4, 5, and 6.

Interpersonal skills training in nurse education

The need to acquire and be able to implement good communication and interpersonal skills has been investigated and documented at some length in the nursing literature. (Porritt, 1984, Faulkner et al., 1983, Kagan, 1985, Burnard, 1985 & 1989, Peplau 1988) Such needs have been translated into

34

curricula aims and objectives which nurse educationalists have been implementing to varying degrees for some years. Much has also been written about the need to integrate theory and practice in nursing (Bendall, 1971, Altschul, 1978, Alexander, 1983) with most of these studies focused on the application of clinical theory to practice within the `general field' (now called the Registered General Nursing field). Some studies have looked at how communication skills and interpersonal skills taught in Colleges of Nursing have been applied to patient care, for example, Altschul (1980), Ashworth (1980), Kagan (1985), Tomlinson (1988) among others. Other studies investigated interpersonal skills as `management of people skills' from a hierarchical perspective, such as ward managers with learners (Fretwell 1978, Ogier 1980, Porritt 1984, and Skevington 1984) but little substantial work has been done on how nurses used these interpersonal skills for their own benefit, although they can be seen in studies looking at the socialisation of nurses. (Kincey and Kat 1984, Hayman and Shaw 1984, Melia 1987 and Smith 1992)

The rationale for teaching communication and interpersonal skills can be found in the many publications in the nursing literature on the subject. Good communication and interpersonal skills are advocated in nursing curricula as a result of the research findings of those listed above as well as other seminal work done, for example Ashworth (1980) in intensive care nursing, Wilson-Barnett (1978) in communication with patients (prior to invasive investigation), Maguire (1985), Macleod-Clark (1985) on the consequences of poor communication between nurses and patients and the Communication in Nurse Education project (C.I.N.E. project) by Tomlinson (1988), Burnard & Morrison (1988) and others studying the quality of nurses' communication skills. Poor communication between nurses and patients has been highlighted from diverse sources; from formal complaints to the ombudsman about the consequence of poor communication. These complaints ranged from minor forms of poor communication to serious incidents which demonstrated a degree of neglect of patients while under the care of medical and nursing staff that often went unpublished (Ley 1972, 1982). Examples of good communication are not so obvious in the literature, perhaps because it is taken for granted and only recognised as deficient when patients or others experience adverse consequences of communication, a point well made by Fielding and Llewelyn (1987) when they spoke of the UK cultural deep suspicion about communication. However, some patients have written about their good experiences stating that they measured the quality of nursing care mostly by the quality of the interpersonal relationships nurses bring to their work (Smith, 1992). Many nurse theorists and educators have recommended that the most effective way of developing interpersonal effectiveness is through training in self-awareness, assertiveness and stress management (Burnard, 1991). These interpersonal skills would facilitate the nurse developing healthy options for managing the complexity of the occupational role, (Townsend, 1983b, Burnard,

1985, 1990, Kagan, 1985, Marson, 1985, Bond, 1986, Kagan et al., 1986, Bond & Kilty, 1990 and Barber, 1993). In spite of the fact that so many studies have been done and published in the nursing literature about the nurse-patient relationship, few studies have looked at how nurses use communication and therapeutic interpersonal skills to explore in themselves the full intensity of his or her selfhood and their relationship which is the primary aim of humanistic experiential education. Kagan (1985) refers to this when she reflects on the need for nurses and tutors to develop skills of working co-operatively together as such skills are essential for nursing practice. She goes on to say:

> It is unhelpful for nurses to employ "all" their interpersonal skills
> effectively when relating to patients, but then to go on to be curt and
> dismissive to colleagues. Patients can be made to feel very
> uncomfortable if they overhear such encounters, and staff morale may
> well be affected (with its attendant consequences for patients). (Kagan,
> 1985, p291)

From the above it would seem that nurses may need to make fundamental changes to how they relate to others rather than just using interpersonal skills as `behavioural repertoire' to use `on' patients.

The S.O.N.(1) curriculum for the interpersonal skills strand was very comprehensive with the intention that students be holistically educated in therapeutic interpersonal relating. Throughout the curriculum the communication and interpersonal skills are clinical context related, however, whether these skills as personal qualities deepen either experientially or theoretically is not clear, either as an educational intention or in practice.

Conclusion

This Chapter has provided the background of this research from my personal biography, to the interpersonal nature of nursing and has looked at the philosophical perspective underpinning the educational and clinical practice of nursing. The need to explore the definition of nursing which could give a theoretical framework to the interpersonal relationships among nurses was found within the humanistic conceptual framework and from there humanistic approaches to the education of adults, particularly professional education, naturally followed. Most significantly, the definition of the educated person from Heron (1974) was offered as a `standard' by which (professional) educational outcomes for individuals and nurses as a social group could be assessed. The educated person is one who can use self, their presence and their interpersonal skills to benefit self and others. This belief is the basis for the interpersonal skills strand in nurse educational curricula and for the approaches advocated to teach it. For educated people are as competent emotionally as they are intellectually and behaviourally and are as cognisant of their beliefs and values as they are of the psychomotor skills they need for their work. To access learning at an emotional, values and belief level experiential learning approaches are advocated and it was the problems associated with attempting to apply such teaching practices which initiated this research.

Notes

1   It is necessary to explain how the different venues where the experiences an where the research took place have been coded, as these are the same location. (See also Chapter 3) The first School of Nursing is codes S.O.N (1). When this S.O.N. was in a transitional phase of amalgamation with another School of Nursing the code is S.O.N.(2) and when the final amalgamation took place both Schools became a College of Nursing which is sometimes abbreviated to C.O.N. (1).

2   Experiential learning is learning which actively involves the learner and where learning comes from concrete experience. (Weil & McGill, 1989, p.174)

3   'Enabling as I will use in incorporates Roger's notion of empathy, positive regard and genuineness, as well as the dictionary definition of 'to authorise, empower a person to take certain actions' (Oxford English Dictionary 1982)

4   Therapeutic means curative, of the healing art. Actions of remedial agents in disease or health. (Oxford English Dictionary 1982) Therapeutic implies an intention to facilitate healing in mind, body and spirit if nursing is holistic.

5   Participative or interactive teaching methods include experiential exercises, critical incidence analysis, debates, seminars and role-playing techniques in interpersonal skills training

2 Research philosophy and methodology

Introduction

In this chapter a brief exposition of the research philosophy of constructivism and its place within the broader research field will be given. The constructivist ontological (fundamental assumptions about the nature of existence, of reality) and epistemological (assumptions about the nature of knowledge) bases will be explored. This will demonstrate that the methodology (the theory of how methods work) and the methods chosen are internally congruent within the chosen paradigm. Tosey defines the term paradigm comprehensively when he says:

> A paradigm is a constellation of beliefs and values and related metaphors, models and practices. A paradigm is an underlying, fundamental worldview, in many ways tacit, so that it leads us to perceive and interpret our world in particular ways without us necessarily being aware of the assumptions we are making. (Tosey, 1993, p.17)

The methodology used will be described in some detail, mainly to illustrate how the systematic inquiry was conducted using appropriate methods to achieve the research purpose and to demonstrate the emergence of a substantive theory. The research methods will be covered in Chapter 3 and examples of data coding and categorisation can be found in Appendix B.

The choice of a constructivist paradigm

The impetus to conduct this research using a constructivist paradigm was borne out of my wish to explore in a systematic way what it is like for nurses relating to other nurses within the work setting. Aspiring nurses come together to a college of nursing to form a learning group and go through intense educational and working relationships for a three year period which then sets the scene for professional working relations. The intensive learning and working relationships seem 'taken for granted' as part of being a nurse, and preparing to be a nurse. The educational and working goal for nurses is to give high quality caring to patients and Travelbee (1971), Peplau (1988) and Smith's (1992) studies suggest that nurses are implicitly seeking this same care for themselves. It is the experience of 'caring for and being cared for' that nurses want in their working relationships. Nurses expect of themselves and are expected by others to offer a dedicated professional commitment to giving to other human beings. In that capacity nurses hope to reap job satisfaction, achieve awareness of their own destiny, both personal and professional (Leininger 1985) and, according to Melia's (1987) study, hope to have the necessary physical and emotional strength to meet the demands of the job they have chosen.

The world of nursing is in the main a social, subjective world (Munhall and Oiler 1986, xii) of human needs embracing physical, mental, emotional and spiritual health and illness. Nurses frequently engage in activities which touch on human vulnerability, dependency and interdependency through intimate contact with physical, emotional and social events of significance to themselves and to their clients. This research sought to understand the subjective meanings that nurses give to their experiences, firstly in an effort to identify some of the elements of interpersonal relationships between nurses themselves which are raised by such experiences; secondly, to link this with the educational processes about interpersonal relations; and thirdly, to find out how such issues are addressed as part of educating people for the work of nursing.

Remembering that the research questions posed in Chapter 1 were:

1   What are your interpersonal relationships like, with each other as students, with tutors, and with ward staff?

2   Personal and interpersonal skills training is part of nurse education. How might such training raise personal and interpersonal issues for you, both in the School of Nursing and on the wards?

the research paradigm needed to be one which would yield answers to these questions by allowing the research participants to explore their working and educational interpersonal relationships, particularly encouraging them to share their beliefs and values about such interpersonal experiences. The methodology needed to be such as to enable analyse of participants' constructions and re-constructions of experiences to give an accurate understanding and interpretation of subjective accounts. As Denzin postulates:

> Subjective experience involves drawing on personal experience or the personal experience of others in an effort to form an understanding and interpretation of particular phenomena. Objective knowledge assumes that

one can stand outside an experience and understand it, independent of the persons experiencing the phenomenon in question. Intersubjective knowing rests on shared experiences and the knowledge gained from having participated in a common experience with another person. (Denzin 1984, p.133)

The concept of intersubjectivity is significant for qualitative research as it stands in place of any claim for 'objective reality' in traditional social science. (Lincoln and Guba, 1985, p.292) Denzin elaborates this intersubjectivity in a further publication when he says that:

Such understanding rests on an interpretative process that leads one to enter into the emotional life of another. Interpretation, the act of interpreting and making sense out of something, creates the conditions for understanding, which involves being able to grasp the meanings of an interpreted experience for another individual. Understanding is an intersubjective emotional process. Its goal is to build sharable understandings of the life experience of another...this is creating verisimilitude or truth-like intersubjectively sharable emotional feelings and cognitive understandings. (Denzin, 1989, pp.27-28)

Thus the intention in using a constructivist approach for this study was to develop an intersubjective knowing of the interpersonal dynamic between nurses, that is, to ascertain the interpersonal processes at play when they engage in their work and learning. That nurses are expected to relate to each other as part of nursing is shown by one of the curricular aims:

The Nurses will use appropriate communication skills, develop therapeutic relationships with patients, carers and other members of the health care team in order to initiate and sustain continuity of care until optimum independence is achieved. (S.O.N.(1) 1989)

There are multiple realities for individuals or epistemic styles, that is, distinctive personal ways of knowing; rational, empirical, and metaphorical. Skevington (1984) talks of the multiple perspectives within the social situations of work such as the social systems approach, which looks at role requirements within the overall structure and functions within the organisation, and the interactionist approach where relationships are juxtaposed between the aims of nursing, the health care structure (patient focused) and the individual needs of nurses.

In the interactionist approach negotiation of mutual expectations in concrete situations is the central aspect of interpersonal relationships. (Skevington, 1984, p.38)

41

It is pertinent to gather information from all those involved in the experience to know how they are being effective and achieving what they think their role and function is. This type of inquiry is of the hermeneutic phenomenological style which is a method of finding out the 'correct interpretation' from many different sources, for:

> All understanding is hermeneutical, taking place, and to a large extent determined by, our finite existence in time, history and culture... we are historical beings, and our understanding is a historical process. (Rowan, 1981, p132)

The importance of seeing connected patterns between different peoples' world realities will give an idea of commonality (Kelly 1955), of the collective unconscious (Jung 1971), and of the basic sociopsychological processes (Glaser & Strauss 1967) operating in groups and the social systems (institutions) in which they function (Berger & Luckmann 1971). The methodology of grounded theory draws on all these conceptual frameworks by its methods of data collecting, its systematic analysis of data, (seeking individual and collective social patterns) using the 'verstehen' approach and its focus on generating theory about social processes. This matched my research intention which was to place emphasis on 'illumination, understanding and extrapolation from data, all techniques encouraged in the constructivist approach, rather than look for causal determination, prediction and generalisation'. (Patton, 1990, p.424)

The constructivist paradigm

Practitioners of the constructivist approach believe that knowledge is actually constructions of reality (Pope and Denicolo 1986) and that these realities must be seen as a 'whole picture' which cannot be understood in isolation from their context. The context needs to include the experience which the observer brings to every new situation in the light of conceptual models built up from past experiences. The research interaction should take place with the entity-in-context for fullest understanding. Lincoln and Guba (1985) explain this when they say:

> Context is crucial in deciding whether or not a finding may have meaning in some other context as well (Lincoln and Guba, 1985, p.38).

What this means in practice is that deliberate freezing out of some of the social contexts or the controlling of variables could impoverish interpretation of the whole social scene. As well as the holist view expressed above, the anthropomorphic model of man would argue that individuals are social beings and self-controlling agents. This belief also reinforces the notion that, 'interpretation of personal reports needs to be done within a social context'. (Harré and Secord, 1972, p.38). This study is about social relationships and behaviour, and therefore the events must be connected to concepts which are appropriate to the descriptions of the social reality as described by those in the situation. There are many ways within social science of finding out about people's perceptions, beliefs and values; about what they think they need and how they relate to others in their social world. In constructivist inquiry, with its different methodologies, the singular characteristic which unites them all is reflected in Kelly's (1955) notion of 'If you want to know what is going on for an individual, ask him'. This implies that the person in the experience is the only authentic source of knowledge of that person's reality. According to Denzin (1989):

> Persons as selves have experiences, experiences referring here to the individuals meeting, confronting, passing through, and making sense of events in their lives. (Denzin, 1989, p.33)

In recognising that social phenomena are constructed from the understandings and meanings that people bring to the social situation, constructivist inquirers would see that such constructions of reality would determine the behaviour adopted (Field and Morse 1985). This philosophical assumption was encapsulated in Kelly's (1955) fundamental postulate:

> A person's processes are psychologically channelised by the ways in which they anticipate events. (Bannister & Francella, 1986, p.7)

Thus this research assumes that the way the person gives meaning to sense-impressions markedly influences his/ her feelings, thoughts and actions. Giving meaning to sense-impressions or experience is done by a combination of perceptual awareness, a 'from to' knowing or tacit knowledge (Polanyi and Prosch, 1975, p.34) and by a combination of propositional knowledge, (assertions of facts) with experiential (face-to-face encounter in the experience) and practical knowledge (Heron, 1981, p.27). All these forms of knowledge are embraced within a constructivist paradigm.

Applying the constructivist paradigm

In posing the question: How can this research be most effectively carried out? The answer lay in taking account of the important dimension of subjective interpretation. This approach is referred to as Interpretative Sociology and is the foundation stone of the naturalistic approach (Denzin 1989). The naturalist researcher within Interpretative Sociology, seeks to understand the 'other's world' by combining 'the other's' interpretative framework with their own for the purpose of describing, interpreting, and offering tentative hypotheses about the social processes under scrutiny (Schutz, 1967, p.11). To this end, constructivists lean towards dialectic methods (Reason and Rowan 1981) of data collecting and analysis. By dialectic is meant `a comparison and contrast of various views with the aim of achieving a higher-level synthesis of individual constructions' (Guba and Lincoln, 1989, p.149)

The constructivist paradigm has travelled historically under the name of `naturalistic inquiry' as well as other aliases, for example: postpositivistic, hermeneutic or interpretive paradigms informing many methodologies, such as, ethnographic, phenomenological, case study, qualitative, or humanistic (co-operative) inquiry (Lincoln and Guba, 1985, p.7 and 1989, p.83). The core value shared by all these different perspectives is the respect for the individual perceptions, their self-determinism and their ability to interpret and articulate their own realities. The two main features of the constructivist approach are:

(1)   that the researcher gets as close as possible to the natural setting in which the actors play their social role(s), and

(2)   that any emerging hypothesis or theory derives from the people being studied and in co-operation with them. That is, there are no preconceived and predetermined `truths' to be tested out and therefore no manipulations of the research field on the part of the researcher. (adapted from Lincoln and Guba, 1985, p.8).

The constructivist paradigm is termed postpositivist (Lincoln and Guba, 1989) as a way of differentiating it from the more traditional prepositive natural science (passive observer-approach) and more particularly from the positivist (active interventionist) natural and social science / human science approach to research. (Schwartz and Ogilvy 1979). The need to define differently the development of substantive (discipline) thought and the shift from a positivist to a postpositivist stance is justified:

For, if a new paradigm of thought and belief is emerging, it is necessary to construct a parallel new paradigm of inquiry (Lincoln and Guba, 1985, p.16).

The differences in beliefs which guide methodologies between the positivist and postpositivist paradigm areas can be summed up in the following way; the positivistic paradigm embraces and works with the working postulates of materialism, reductionism, dealing with universal laws and issues of quantification, predictions, neutrality and objectivity. The postpositivist (constructivist) paradigm gives as a framework concepts of multiple perspectives and individual perception; it is inductivist, looking for emerging patterns-qualification, allowing for subjectivity in interpretation, respects human values, and aims at context integration. (Munhall & Oiler 1986) In these salient points of differences in beliefs can be seen the internal consistency which is essential to hold within a paradigm for 'congruence of axioms (beliefs) and how these inform epistemological, methodological and interpretative frameworks. (Munhall and Oiler, 1986)

Within the constructivist paradigm the methodology is hermeneutic, that is interpretive in character. (Guba and Lincoln, 1989, p.149) Approaching fieldwork without imposing pre-determined categories of analysis allows for a more open, indepth and detailed dialectic (qualitative) inquiry. The importance of tacit knowledge (Polanyi 1966), experiential and practical knowledge (Heron 1981), guiding and informing the research is valued as befits an emic approach. Equally, the interpretative explanation of qualitative analysis does not yield knowledge in the same way as quantitative explanation. As stated earlier (Patton, 1990, p.424) the emphasis in qualitative research is on illumination, understanding and extrapolation rather than causal determination, prediction and generalisation which are characteristics of conventional (quantitative) methods.

The positivist (conventional) approach requires the use of standardised measures so that the varying perspectives and experiences of people can fit into a limited number of predetermined response categories to which numbers are assigned. (Patton, 1990, p.14) The advantage of the conventional approach is that it allows for the measurement of reactions of many people to a limited set of questions to give a broad, generalisable set of findings presented succinctly and parsimoniously. Quantitative methodologies known as the traditional scientific approach are based on deductive reasoning, objectivity, and theory testing using quasi-experimental, statistical techniques with control of variables for the most part. (Reichardt and Cook 1979)

For this study, it is not the intention to critique the different paradigms or methodologies to decide which is better, but rather to say that both have their place in research, depending on the purpose of the research (Hammersley and Atkinson, 1983, p.x). Light and Pillemer (1982, p.19) speak of an 'Alliance of evidence' that finds its origin in qualitative idiographic research (for describing what is new and for theory generation) and its validation (verification and generalisability) in quantitative nomothetic research. However this distinction is artificial as in the constructivist paradigm 'discovery and verification are continuous interactive processes (Guba and Lincoln, 1989, p.182).

Of the many perspectives under the umbrella of the constructivist paradigm: phenomenology, ethnography, ethnomethodology, action research, indepth case study and grounded theory, the last, grounded theory, was chosen for this study. This choice was based on a preference to study the 'inner' or experiential aspects of people in the form of their encounters with their experience, their perceptions and beliefs and link that experience with the social world with which the individual interacts. As Strauss & Corbin (1990, p.159) stated, 'grounded theory is a transactional system, that is, it allows you to study the interactive nature of events'. The specific advantages of this approach will be discussed in the next section. Also, the rigour and quality of its theoretical analysis and theory generation is

45

challenging. Added to this is the evidence of such works as Glaser & Strauss (1965), Chenitz & Swanson (1986), Munhall & Oiler (1986), Melia (1987), Cowley (1991) and Smith (1992) among others who used grounded theory within a health care / social setting and whose results were stimulating and relevant to the nursing profession.

The research methodology - grounded theory

Along with the various descriptions of grounded theory drawn from academic researchers in the field, there will by my own experiential understanding of the approach which helped me conclude that grounded theory is a research methodology which has a distinctive set of analytical processes and product. The processes of grounded theory move the analyst through and beyond descriptive data, by systematic theoretical inquiry of *what is going on in the data and how it is being manifested,* to theoretical interpretation from that data of social and psychosocial aspects of human experience. The product of grounded theory is the generation of hypotheses or the development of a tentative theory about social phenomena.

The theoretical foundation of grounded theory is based on the Symbolic Interactionist perspective where the symbols which people use, whether they are objects or acts, have meaning and value for the users. Symbolic Interactionism holds three main premises, which are:

1   Human beings act toward things on the basis of the meanings that the thing has for them;

2   the meaning of such things is derived from, or arises out of the social interaction that one has with one's fellows; and

3   meanings are handled in, and modified through, an interpretive process and by the person dealing with the things he encounters (Blumer, 1969, p.2).

Symbols such as clothes, verbal and non-verbal language, social constructs and other artifacts are ways of presenting self to the world (Stern et al., 1982, p.203). Grounded theory aims to examine social interactions in their symbolic form for the purpose of description and theory generation at a local level (Elden 1981). As Atwood & Hinds defined it: 'The ultimate purpose of grounded theory is to generate a series of hypotheses that then define the social process' (Atwood and Hind, 1986, p.136). This method of `discovering theory from data' was first developed by the sociologists Glaser and Strauss (1965) in the course of their studies of American health care institutions. According to Strauss:

> Grounded theory is based on a concept indicator model which directs the conceptual coding of a set of empirical indicators (Strauss, 1987, p.25).

The data are what people say or do and which the analyst draws out and gives a concept label. The relationship between the indicators of the concept and the concept itself is best illustrated by Strauss (1987, p.25) himself:

Figure 2.1. Indicator-concept model

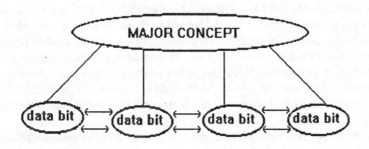

Chenitz and Swanson (1986, p.3) define grounded theory as:

> ..a naturalistic science gaining its reputation by the sophisticated way it handles qualitative data gathered in the natural, everyday world. It is a rigorous systematic approach of data collecting and analysis to study fundamental patterns known as basic social-psychological processes which account for variation in interaction within a given setting or problem for the purpose of generating explanatory theory that furthers the understanding of social and psychological phenomena.

Grounded theory can be presented either as well codified sets of propositions or in a running theoretical discussion using conceptual categories and their properties following Glaser and Strauss' (1967, p.31) description. As Kalpin (1964, p.296) explains:

> Theoretical concepts are contrasted with observational ones, and theoretical laws with empirical generalisations. Though all conception involves the use of symbols and is thereby distinguished from perception, in some cases the symbols relate directly to the perceptual materials while in other cases the relation is mediated by still further symbolic processes.

Grounded theory can be used to research a specific substantive 'local' area of inquiry, or it can develop into a formal 'grand' theory addressing the conceptual level of inquiry of social processes, such as status passage, socialisation, stigma. (Hutchinson 1986). The research process has many distinct stages, (Turner 1981, Munhall and Oiler 1986, Atwood and Hinds 1986, Strauss 1987) although how one follows the stages, in what depth and in what manner is a decision left to the individual researcher. Glaser & Strauss, like other grounded theorists after them, for example Turner (1981), have not wanted to be dogmatic in prescribing a 'one right way' which they deemed to be part of the positivistic mode. The stages will be briefly described here as part of the general description of grounded theory, and in Chapter 3 the stages will be explained in more detail as they were applied in this research.

Grounded theory aims to generate theory from data systematically obtained and analysed from social research. However one needs to find out what is happening in relation to something. For this research this meant finding out what was happening:

♦　　　　in relation to the interpersonal dynamic among nurses in the work setting,
♦　　　　in relation to interpersonal skills education and how this was supported by ward staff and applied in practice.

This ability of grounded theory to focus on relational dimensions as units of analysis fitted the requirements for an approach which would allow the examination of experience and assumptions about the interpersonal relationships of nurses at work. It also allows for the examination of the educational influence on interpersonal relating within the School of Nursing as well as their relevance and effectiveness for nurses in relating at a personal and professional level. As stated earlier in this chapter, exploring people's perceptions is to move into a complex, subjective reality of individual world views, and also to move to a collective reality as people influence each other's values, beliefs and behaviour. To access such perceptions needs indepth unstructured inquiry. Equally, to interpret from the data and to make predictions and recommendations needs the co-operation and confirmation of finding by the informants if the interpretations are to have any validity in the social context from which the data arose.

Grounded theory 'must meet four central criteria for judging the applicability of theory to a phenomenon. These are: *fit, understanding, generality,* and *control*' (Strauss & Corbin, 1990, p.23). If these criteria are met then the analysis of data should provide clear enough concepts and hypotheses so that salient categories can be verified in present and future research. The emerging theory must *fit* the situation being researched, and *work* when put into use. Glaser & Strauss were very particular about this when they said:

> By 'fit' is meant that the category must be readily, (not forcibly) applicable to and indicated by the data under study; by 'work' is meant that they must

be meaningfully relevant to and be able to explain the behaviour under study (Glaser and Strauss 1967, p. 22)

That is, the data and the analysis must be understood by both the researcher and the participants alike. However, if the conceptualisation is abstract and broad then some generality would be appropriate, yet keeping the findings context related within the area of study where it was found; here lies the control.

In writing about accuracy, they go on to say:

> In grounded theory, it is not the fact by which we stand, but the conceptual category (or a conceptual property of the category) that was generated from it. Accuracy is not at stake as much as establishing the structural boundaries of a fact (Glaser and Strauss, 1967, p.23).

In grounded theory the research questions take the form of:

a   What is going on in the data?
b   What are these data a study of?
c   What is the basic socio-psychological process / problem with which these people must deal?
d   What basic socio-psychological processes help them to cope with the problem?

These questions become more specific and systematic when the six `C's are used. (Glaser 1978, see page 52) Having identified the likely basic social processes the researcher then focuses the enquiry onto incidents which confirm or reject the basic social process or modifies it. Theory is derived from the data and then illustrated by characteristic examples of data. These questions would form part of the hermeneutic dialectic inquiry stated in an earlier section of this chapter.

The use of the literature in grounded theory

The place of the literature review in grounded theory is effectively to place the research in the context under study. In the initial phases of the study the literature can be used to set the scene (as in Chapter 1 of this report). However it is advocated that using a literature review to search out conceptual frameworks with which to interpret incoming data is contrary to the theory generating process of grounded theory. (Glaser 1978, Stern 1985, Becker 1993). Stern (1985) goes so far as to list three main disadvantages to a pre-study literature review, these are:

♦   The search may lead to prejudgment and effect premature closure of ideas and research inquiry;
♦   The direction may be wrong; and

♦   The available data or materials used may be inaccurate (ibid., 1985, p.153)

These are strong warnings which need to be heeded if the researcher is actively to engage in theory generation rather than theory confirmation. Glaser is so adamant about this that he encourages the researcher:

> To *read in other areas'* rather than the one under study until all the first coding, memos, sorting of memos and some firm integration of findings *(has occurred)* so as not to preempt thoughts regarding the significant variables in the substantive area under research. (Glaser, 1978, p.139)

This advice seemed well founded, as the temptation to jump into premature logical theoretical build on flimsy evidence was very real.

Glaser (1978) and Stern (1985) among others do encourage exploring the literature for descriptive accounts in the general area of study, particularly where there is little interpretation as this helps theoretical sensitivity and in effect can act as part of theoretical sampling. Some of the studies by other researchers have been used in this way in this study. During the consolidation of theoretical categories and the writing of the thesis drafts then it is important, according to Glaser, to use the existing literature in the area of study for the:

> ..purpose of comparing your findings with that of others and to integrate your theory with others to build a theoretical and substantive literature. (ibid., 1978, p.139)

The stages of grounded theory

The nine stages of grounded theory listed below in an adapted summary from Turner (1981, p.231) after Glaser and Strauss (1967). These stages were used as guidelines for dealing with the complexity of data handling in grounded theory. The reason for choosing Turner's work was that it seemed the most succinct description of the methodology, geared to meeting the needs of `new grounded researchers' without getting `bogged down' in the theoretical expositions found in many research books. The descriptions also take into account other authors' expert views (Munhall and Oiler 1986, Chenitz and Swanson 1986) on the method and my own understanding of grounded theory as I applied it in this research.

Stage 1 Develop categories

Initial interviews and observations are used to spread a wide net to gather as much relevant data as possible about the phenomena under study. Sampling is usually purposeful to select information-rich cases for indepth studies. (Patton, 1990, p.182)

Identifiable relational units of analysis are sorted into substantive codes, paragraph by paragraph, and provisional labels or categories assigned to them. The label or category needs to be a conceptual one, possessing one essential property, ie, it must 'fit' the phenomenon described in the data (Turner, 1981, p.232). As Turner emphasised, correct fit forms the basis of subsequent operations. This was re-informed by Swanson when she said:

> Glaser (1978) defined categories and their characteristics (properties) as conceptual codes depicting the essential relationship between data and theory. They are building blocks to theory and are important for description and initial analysis of qualitative data. (Swanson, 1986, p.122)

Corbin also defines a category as:

> a conceptualisation of several similar incidents or concepts, which at the early stages still needs to be more fully developed and densified by discovering its properties, the conditions under which it occurs and how it is manifested. (Corbin, 1986, p.95)

The building blocks are developed by theoretical coding. Strauss and Corbin are at pains to point out that 'coding' *is* the analysis of data. They go on to say:

> Coding represents the operations by which data are broken down, conceptualised, and put back together in new ways. (Strauss and Corbin, 1990, p.57)

This theoretical coding enables the researcher to step back from the data and look at the relationships between codes and categories. Questions asked of the data are based on the six "C" devised by Glaser (1978) to explore and explain the conceptual linkages of codes towards theory building. These six 'C's are:

Cause, Consequences, Conditions, Context, Contingencies, Co-variances

---

which according to Glaser (1978: 74) are the 'bread and butter' of theoretical analysis for social phenomena. Questions are asked of the data, such as:

- What causes this phenomenon to occur?
- What are the conditions for its emergence, significance and stability over time?
- How does one substantive category link with others?
- In what way does this category co-vary with another?
- What are the context, the contingencies and so on.

The rigour with which the researcher asks and answers these questions is analogous to quantitative measurement, that is:

> In grounded theory, measurement is the process of linking concepts to data bits or transcending the data to achieve theoretical abstractness (Atwood and Hinds, 1986, p.137).

This process of rigorous inquiry occurs in Stage 2 as part of the constant comparative analysis.

Stage 2 Saturate categories

Once categories have been identified, however crudely, further examples are sought for in the data, in further interviews and by going back to the fieldwork as necessary to look for incidents of the category. The categories at this stage can be low conceptual level categories or descriptive in nature. Elements of the category are identified and new phenomena are included or excluded according to identified elements. This is referred to as 'constant comparative analysis', a concept developed by Glaser and Strauss (1967). The main method for doing this is through a systematic process called theoretical memoing which is a written record of the thoughts in the form of questions, ideas, theoretical linkage which went on in the researcher's mind as s/he worked through the data and coding process. According to Corbin (1986) these theoretical memos are researcher-imposed meanings on the data and form the beginnings of analytical strategies and theory formation (ibid., 1986, pp.102-120).

It is from comparative analysis that theory development, saturation, verification and conclusions are drawn.

Stage 3 Abstract definitions

Consolidating the categories is done by a more abstract definition of the concepts and categories. The need to reach theoretical saturation based on data rich in definition, that is, indepth exploration of all the elements of a phenomenon, with succinct examples from the data to illustrate the definition, is important to create a dense emerging grounded theory.

Categories may be simple relational units of analysis, or there may be many properties of the category, with many sub-processes under a major complex category. Some of the properties may overlap, linking with other processes and other categories which is more likely the further away from the raw data one moves to core categories. Theoretical abstraction moves further into the core category / categories which explains the *basic sociopsychological process* that the person or group is dealing with over time. The purpose of categories and the hierarchical linking of categories is to:

get to those *basic sociopsychological processes* which are relevant and problematic for those involved. (Glaser, 1978, p.93)

and

The core category needs to be able to embrace all other categories in the study at the same time to allow for greater generalisability. (Chenitz and Swanson, 1986, p.13)

Stage 4 Use the definition

Once the definitions have been clarified, further incidents can be assigned to the category. The researcher is sensitised to `spot' the processes of the category, or the category-in-action. Whereas earlier they might have done this intuitively, now the veils have lifted and they can articulate the processes and broaden their horizons to see the same processes going on in other contexts. The original data has helped build the category; now the category in its theoretical form is at a higher level of abstraction and therefore no longer dependent on the original raw data.

Stage 5 Exploit categories

Exploiting categories is related to Glaser's (1978) *theoretical sampling,* when the researcher tests out the categories in other situations or if necessary with other groups to check for their existence and their robustness. Seeking the `negative case' is a valid method of testing the validity of categories (Strauss and Corbin, 1990, pp.108-109). Non-existence of a phenomenon (basic social process) in different social/ cultural environments re-enforces the validity in terms of variety in different contexts and is to be valued. Tentative predictions can be formulated and tested out. This process is essentially a conceptual elaboration, that is, being able `to read' processes at different levels of abstraction, in different contexts and being able to `see' theoretical links at the social-psychological level which on the surface seemed quite dissimilar.

Saliency

Saliency is a significant factor throughout coding, category formation and comparative analysis. The frequency and intensity with which a particular concept is repeated over and over again and in different situations, shows it to be a robust concept; equally significant, absence of a concept from some data needs to be acknowledged and accounted for. In the following examples of analysis of raw data, the salient factors may seem hidden in the process codes. However, when drawing up the taxonomies of hierarchical categories they become more obvious. Salient categories that illuminate social phenomena such as `awareness of dying, closed awareness or open awareness' (Glaser and Strauss, 1965) are labelled the basic social process (or problem) which the people in the study are managing either effectively or not.

Stages 1 to 5 illustrate a difficult balance for the research between the raw data from respondents and its relevance to the area under study. In putting out a wide net to 'catch' what might be significant elements of an emerging theory, the chances of collecting more than can be analysed, and analysing data that is tangential from the main unit of analysis is quite high. It will be seen that such a danger was encountered in this study. The other main danger is that the researcher may impose his/ her frame of reference on the data.

Turner (1981) does not refer explicitly to the terms 'theoretical coding' or 'theoretical memos', yet these were Glaser and Strauss' (1967) main way of teasing out underlying processes, both social and psychological, which enabled verbal and behavioural descriptions to be raised to theoretical concepts for the purpose of hypothesising and theory building.

Stage 6   Develop and follow-up links between categories

Relational diagrams in the form of hierarchical taxonomies are created. This helps to illustrate the possible causal properties linking theoretical concepts. The purpose of the diagrams is to identify the most salient core categories and ultimately a central core category or basic sociopsychological process which subsumes and accounts for all the processes going on in the data.

Stage 7   Consider the conditions under which the links hold

This is an extension of Stage 6 and looks at conditions under which outcomes occur; why one particular outcome occurs over another when analysed using the six 'C's. as recommended by Glaser (1978, p.74)

Stage 8   Make connections where relevant, to existing theory

The researcher can inform her /himself about the categories by referring to the literature with respect to content, interpretation and application. This is a different way of using existing theory, as the researcher has already developed propositions from his/her own data and goes to the existing theory to see if it has anything useful to offer. Emerging theory develops with more diagramming, more linkage and more sorting of data that was put to one side. As Turner (1981) explains, 'the process aims to crystallise the emerging relational clusters from which a theoretical statement is produced, however crudely'. In summary, Turner states that in terms of rigour, categories must have:

1   A closeness of fit, that is, that those in the situation under study can readily
         recognise the phenomena or the basic sociopsychological processes.
         Negotiating mutual understanding between researcher and participants is
         an important part of grounded theory, as it purports to interpret their
         perceptions in generating categories and emerging theory.

2 .   A degree of complexity. When studying social phenomena, particularly if
         the focus is to develop formal theory, the emerging theory needs to reflect
         the multi-dimensional aspects of the world these people live in. (Adapted
         from Turner, 1981, p.240).

Stage 9   Use extreme comparisons to the maximum to test emerging relations

This stage is an extension of Stage 5 but with more emphasis on finding the central
proposition or core category:

> ..while process (a basic sociopsychological process) is always a core
> category, not all core categories are process categories. In a grounded
> theory study, a core category always exists; however a basic social process
> does not (Fagerhaugh, 1986, p.135).

The basic socio-psychological processes and other core processes form the material
for propositional statements. It is here that an emerging personal and social
epistemology is formulated, that is a theoretical interpretation at an individual and
social level is made. The emerging categories are shared with the participants for
confirmation of the findings with respect to the interpretation the researcher offers
of the data. Glaser and Strauss (1967) saw this sharing as a measure of face validity,
that is, seeking reactions from participants in the study to ascertain whether they
recognised the researcher's interpretation as fitting with their own. Also, sharing
with peers for debriefing as advocated by Lincoln and Guba (1985, p.308) and
sharing with academic and professional supervisors who can be supportive as well
as play devil's advocate will not only tease out researcher bias, but act as another
strategy to establish face validity (Atwood and Hinds 1986). As stated earlier, in
grounded theory, generalisability is handled by detailed description during data
collection and assigning membership to a class or unit (building up a category) to
the case under study. External validation rests on internal variety. The greater the
range and the variety sought through theoretical sampling, the more the researcher
can be certain that the data is generalisable to other members of the same class or
units as the phenomenon under study. The greater the internal variety, the greater
the likelihood the rescarcher has sought out and addressed the *`negative case'*, that
is, the case that does not fit an existing category or proposition (Glaser 1978).
    Construct validity emerges out of constant comparative analysis, when all the
properties of the categories are looked for in the context in which they were found

and in other similar contexts which are then made explicit. The properties need to be theoretical variables with their relationship specified. This latter important principle guided this research to see the interpersonal relationship as a dimension and identify it as the unit of analysis for study.

The use of language

The above stages do not explicitly speak about the use of language in research, yet when a researcher goes into the world of others for the purpose of identifying 'what is going on' there is a need to recognise, in terms of the Symbolic Interactionist perspective, a 'mutuality of understanding' (Heron, 1981, p.26) between researcher and participant. Language can be used to good effect or to poor effect in describing and interpreting others' worldviews. Therefore the validation of language to express meaning needs to be by interpersonal experiential knowing (ibid, 1981, p.26). In this research, since reports were given in respondents' language, from which an analysis of conceptual systems were forged, it was important to arrive at a consensus about the meaning of the language being used. This language needed to reflect as accurately as possible the underlying meaning from individual accounts, so that (collective) social meaning could be given to the 'social reality which people in the situation could recognise'. (Harré and Secord, 1972, p.126). Returning to the interviewees with the coded and memoed transcripts to check for clarification and verification was the main way of testing out whether their experiences had been represented fairly and accurately. This went some way towards developing 'common meaning' for the study, as Benoliel stated:

> The meaning of any data collected by man interacting with man must take account of the reality that the investigator relies on a common sense knowledge and everyday language when he selectively notices certain events and makes certain choices about their relevances. (Benoliel, 1975 cit, Wilds, 1992, p.237)

Methods used in grounded theory

To ensure that tentative theory development emerges out of theoretical concepts, grounded theory advocates two main types of data collecting for the purpose of eliciting the world views of others. These are:

1   Intensive interviews
2   observation in the natural setting

As Lincoln and Guba state:

..qualitative methods come more easily to hand when the instrument is a human being... the human-as-instrument is inclined towards methods that are an extension of normal human activities: listening, speaking, reading, and the like. We believe that the human will tend, therefore, towards interviewing, observing, mining available documents and records... (Lincoln and Guba, 1985, p.199).

Indepth intensive interviews

There are two main types of face to face formal interviewing, formal structured interviewing and formal unstructured (intensive) interviewing (Swanson, 1986, p.66). There is also an off-shoot of the formal unstructured interview, which is the informal interview. Lofland and Lofland (1984) call formal unstructured interviews intensive interviews to signal the nature of the interview and the researcher's intentions in such interviews.

They define such an interview as:

> A guided conversation whose goal is to elicit from the interviewee rich, detailed materials that can be used in qualitative analysis. In contrast to "structured interviewing (such as opinion polling) where the goal is to elicit choices between alternative answers to preformed questions on a topic or situation. (ibid., 1984, p.12)

This definition applies equally to unstructured formal and informal interviews (Chenitz, 1986) as the intention of both is 'to go deeply into some aspect of the individual's feelings, motives, attitudes or life history (Jupp and Miller, 1980, p.18). This is why they are called intensive interviewing, and this term will be used to include both in this study. The intensive interview data can be as detailed as the interviewee wants and allows for the person's own words and concepts to explain his/her perceptions and experiences of working with others and the interpersonal dynamics involved. This intensive interview approach allows the informants to reflect deeply on issues which they are normally so immersed in that they find it difficult to stand back and critically review their assumptions and behaviour. This method, combined with relevant observations helps the researcher acquire knowledge of the interviewee's social reality as defined by the interviewee. The purpose of this is to make sure that any interpretation of the data is done within the defined social context, and is recognisable and agreed on by the people in the social setting. The interview itself provides a context that 'gives meaning and structure to the social reality of the interactive process between interviewer and participant'. (Wilde, 1992, p.238) This interactive process means that the data are the result of the dialogue between the participant and interviewer, so the researcher is actively involved in generating the data. Such involvement needs to be acknowledged and accepted as part and parcel of co-operative inquiry. For effective intensive interviewing the researcher needs to have a high level of interpersonal skills and pay attention to all aspects of the interpersonal encounter as defined in Johnson's (1990) model (in Gregory 1994). The difference between the formal and informal unstructured interview is more to do with spontaneity and opportunism on the part of the researcher, who besides doing formal unstructured interviews, uses everyday conversations, social chat and situational questioning as a means of data collecting. Here there is no need to 'make elaborate arrangement for private space, tape recording, or written consent before embarking in social conversation' (Chenitz, 1986, p.80) Provided that those involved know the researcher's identity and intentions which are to use self as action-in-process to conduct the informal interview, then the engagement can happen in whatever social situation is appropriate for data collecting.

The advantages of face to face interviews are that the person being interviewed can stay in control of the process as much as they wish. They may need to be informed of this right as they may give more authority to the researcher than is appropriate. Both parties can seek clarification of language, ideas and concepts used in the discussion. Rapport can be built up, facilitating a deeper awareness and sharing of perceptions by the interviewee. The researcher can follow where the interviewee leads within the boundaries set for the study. The researcher can use the social context of the interview to make comments on the interviewee's behaviour which are either congruent or incongruent with verbal statements, and non-verbal communication so that a valid source of data can be utilised.

The disadvantages of intensive interviewing for this type of research are that the researcher might lead the interviewees down avenues they do not want to go or vice versa. This will happen if both parties do not negotiate the boundaries and power balance within the interview. The researcher might impose her/his own ideas or feelings on the individual being interviewed. The age, gender, social, cultural and professional status of the interviewer might hamper self-disclosure and make the encounter ineffective. The interviewer needs to be very skilled in interview techniques; to build up trust, to facilitate drawing out the interviewee and being both supportive and challenging as appropriate. The authority projected onto the interviewer could impede a more open and honest sharing of professionally unacceptable thinking, feelings and language. Thus taboo subjects might not be spoken about. Because the content of the interviews is not anonymous, that is, they will be used for research purposes, the need to keep the anonymity of the interviewee is paramount. A contract of anonymity needs to be agreed before the research data collecting starts.

Observation in the natural setting

Historically constructivist (naturalistic) inquiry has its roots in anthropology. The urge to immerse oneself in the field of study (where the action is going on) to the point of going native is a known problem for anthropologists. The constructivist inquirer, in this case the grounded theorist, has the same intention as the anthropologist in wanting to find out `What is happening here'. However, the natural setting for grounded theorists is more often the `known' work place, or social/ recreational environment. Such places have their own peculiar culture, social roles, language and behaviour, which are often taken for granted by those who have been socialised into them through professional or social membership. There is much that is hidden within the social milieu which affects beliefs, attitudes and behaviour. Those involved in the social setting may or may not be aware of the sociopsychological processes which direct their energies and behaviour. The role of the grounded theorist is to observe what is happening in the natural setting and reflect back to the participants what she sees. The question of what type of observation, passive or active is crucial, as is the question of how long to stay in the field on a day-by-day basis. There are no hard and fast rules about this as it does depend on the type of data required. However, naturalistic enquirers tend towards prolonged exposure in the field, particularly if it is new to them, so:

> The researcher can learn the context, minimise distortions and build up a good empathic understanding of the people under study and to create trust. (Lincoln and Guba, 1985, p.303)

Participant observation can also help build up evidence to support what people say in informal interviews either by their presence or absence in different situations. However, Lofland and Lofland (1984, p.13) believe the distinction drawn between participant observation and informal intensive interviewing to `be overdrawn and any invidious comparison unwarranted'. They go on to quote from West's (1980, p.39) summary of a review of sociological field reports, that:

> ..the bulk of participant observation data is probably gathered through informal interviews and supplemented by observation.

For this reason, Lofland and Lofland (1984, p.13) stress the `mutuality of participant observation and intensive interviewing as the central techniques of the naturalistic investigator'. In active or participant observation, the advantages are many. They include:

♦ being part of the situation, making one more aware of less tangible social, psychological processes going on, such as people's level of attention; their willingness to help each other; their empathy and level of morale

- The researcher may be seen as more credible for the workers in the field if she takes part in the same activities. However this can have its drawbacks as listed below.

Some of the disadvantages include:

- the researcher may be inclined to go native, that is, become so engrossed in the activity under study that she loses sight of her reason for being there. This form of seduction into an over-sympathetic understanding of the problems of the actors in the scene can seriously distract from maintaining a witnessing role in fieldwork.

- Difficulties in withdrawing from the field to make fieldnotes; these difficulties may be environmental but equally they could be psychological, as participants may see the researcher as a threat, a spy, which may heighten people's sense of insecurity about being watched and reported on. (Davis, 1986, p.54)

To be a passive observer (non-participative) also has its advantages and disadvantages. Advantages include:

- Being free just to observe, with no confusion with participants about your role

- The chances of being more objective as you are not actively engaged with the people or the work you are also trying to observe

- The researcher can move in and out of the field without too much disturbance, so she is more of a free agent and can make and follow her own plan of observation.

The major disadvantages in non-participative (passive) observation are:

- The researcher standing out like ‘a sore thumb', particularly in a culture where the "busy syndrome" is high profile. (Davis, 1986, p.54)

- Participants are more aware that the researcher is there just to observe which may influence their behaviour to a degree which causes the data to be skewed, that is, not natural or usual in that setting

- A lone passive observer is likely to miss more than if two or more researchers were observing together, but the latter is expensive, and time consuming.

60

With regard to both types of observation, the main limitation to this method within a constructivist paradigm is that observation is limited to the external behaviour of those observed with no access to the individual's internal world. Earlier in this chapter it was argued that the main need in this study was to draw on people's subjective experiences as the main source of data for theory generation, therefore observations proved unhelpful.

Whether passive or active, the researcher comes to the situation with his/ her own interpretative frame of reference. This is particularly so if the researcher has previous professional and/ or experiential knowledge of the social setting (that is a nurse researcher or a former patient studying a hospital environment). For this research, rather than try to suspend such knowledge, which is not possible, being aware of, and using such knowledge constructively is a preferred way of working. Spinelli (1987, p.17,) and Heron (1992, p.165) speak of 'bracketing' out preconceptions when acquiring experiential knowledge, so this process can be recommended for field observations, which is experiential knowledge. Although as Heron says:

> ..there is no such thing as an absolutely pristine, stated declaration of what the transaction(s) is really all about. It is at most a revisionary account, set at the frontiers of, and in the context of, the belief systems of the day. There is no way we can avoid the history of our knowledge. (ibid., 1992, p.165)

Triangulation

Within the naturalistic approach, triangulation is encouraged by observation and interpretation of social phenomena from different reflective mirrors. This is usually effected by using different research methods or sources of data to examine the same problem. Denzin (1978, p.28) identified four main triangulation models: 'data triangulation, where a variety of different data sources are used; investigator triangulation, when two or more researchers collect the same data; theory triangulation, the use of different perspectives to make sense of the same data, and methodological triangulation when there is a mixture of paradigms, that is qualitative and quantitative methods used in the research'. Data triangulation was the emphasis in this research, that is, the collection of varied data on the same phenomenon, from different participants, through formal and informal intensive interviewing with some participative observation, done over different phases of fieldwork (Jupp and Miller, 1980) as well as the use of curriculum documents relevant to the study. How these various methods were applied will be the subject of Chapter 3.   However, combined with the data triangulation from the research participants was the hermeneutic (sense-making) process of a dialectical kind where the researcher's perceptions, professional knowledge and experiences were added to those of the participants to further illuminate, understand and extrapolate meaning from the data. In the postpositivist paradigm it is accepted that the knower and the known are inseparable. This applies to research participants, their position as knower and known as well as to the position of the researcher as knower and known and a commitment by both to a joint search for shared understanding. Such an inquiry process might best be understood under the umbrella of the experiential research methodology (Heron 1981). Many feature of experiential research are missing, however, such as joint ownership with the participants of the research topic and research design with separate non-reciprocal relationships. What is similar is the commitment to shared knowledge and experience as appropriate. With this emphasis the experiential research methodology would be defined as weak as participants and researcher are not fully co-researchers. Rowan's (1981: 97-100) dialectical research cycle illustrates the varying degrees of engagement a researcher can have with participants in the research. This model, which can be used within other qualitative methodologies was used in this study as part of the inquiry process within a grounded theory approach.

Conclusion

In this chapter the rationale for selecting a constructivist paradigm was offered with the expressed need to follow a Symbolic Interactionist approach both philosophically and methodologically. The importance of choosing a paradigm that would reflect the researcher's aims about how she wants to encounter the participants in the field was highlighted and discussed. A research which aims to be collaborative, which believes in a relativist ontology with multi-perspectives needs to use the tools which will allow such perspectives to be mirrored as clearly as possible in the data collecting, analysis and reporting. It was seen that grounded theory offered the most flexible yet robust methodology to address the above issues as it allows for both the exploration of individual worldviews and the ability to bring together individual accounts to illuminate social processes of an interpersonal kind within a group. How this can be accomplished was explained using seminal work on methodological issues by Glaser and Strauss (1967) as well as other followers in that field, particularly Turner (1981), Chenitz and Swanson (1986) and more generally Lincoln and Guba (1985, 1989)

It was seen that the purpose of grounded theory was to facilitate description and theory generation at a local level (Elden 1981), so as to generate a series of hypotheses that then define the sociopsychological processes under study, (Atwood & Hind 1986) and have ecological consistency. To fulfil this latter aim, Chapters 3 and appendix B will describe in some detail the application of grounded theory used for this research.

3 Applying grounded theory

Introduction

Initially, as stated in my biography, I hypothesised what might be going on at a psychological level when students seemed very `reluctant' to engage in interpersonal skills training. I thought I might be witnessing social defence mechanisms as described by Menzies (1960) although her accounts had not penetrated the educational processes in any depth and did not deal with the interpersonal relationships amongst nurses per se. As I was dealing with a relatively new area within the nursing curriculum; teaching personal development and interpersonal skills, I decided that rather than act from unsubstantiated assumptions about defence mechanisms, I would investigate `what was going on' in the perceptions of the people involved. In this chapter I intend to explain in some detail the research processes I engaged in to obtain some answers to my questions. As stated in Chapter 2, qualitative research encourages a combination of methods of which observations and intensive interviews are the most popular. The differences between formal and informal intensive interviews were also described, and how this worked in practice will be shown here. The research site documentation used was the School of Nursing (1 or 2) curriculum documents.

Selection of the research site

I based my selection of the research site on my knowledge of the culture of the hospital and School of Nursing (S.O.N. 1) where the research interest first emerged. In total I had worked in this hospital and School of Nursing over a period of five years, from nursing on the wards to teaching (see Personal biography in Chapter 1). I was familiar enough with the nursing practice on many of the wards as well as the teaching practice in the School to have an appreciation of the type of work on the wards and the relationships between tutors in the S.O.N. and the ward staff. I moved from that School of Nursing in 1988 to the Continuing Education Department of an adjacent School of Nursing (S.O.N. 2) which in due course amalgamated with the first. Just before this amalgamation, I had moved to a large College of Nursing in 1989 where I worked for some months before moving into university teaching in 1990. These moves were important in the selection process as I was able to compare different settings when it came to choosing a research location. The small S.O.N (1) had the advantage of more contact between students and tutors, particularly as the students were enrolled for training three times per year in groups (called training sets) of 24 or fewer, and they were the responsibility of one tutor for the duration of their training. All students had contact with most of the other tutors as the teaching of specialist subjects was shared among the tutors. More importantly, about 4-6 students per training set were allocated to a personal tutor for their academic and personal guidance which allowed for more contact between tutors and students. So with eight tutors and about 240 students at various stages of their training there was enough diversity and also enough familiarity for some form of relationship to develop between tutors and students. Smaller groups seem to find it easier to relate to each other and in fact group sizes comprising 16 to 24 are a large group, (Jaques 1991). However, there was still the possibility of relationships forming which would be of benefit to this research. My short experience in the large College of Nursing in 1989 showed a different pattern. Here large groups of students (30 plus), entered the college once per year. The students were dispersed over a wide geographical area for their ward experiences with ill-defined relationships with college staff. The larger college of nursing would not have been suitable because:

- I was in a senior management position, and rapport with tutors and students would have been more difficult because of the hierarchical power
- the relationships boundaries between students and tutors were tenuous.
- relationships on the wards were also more difficult to define because the wards were specialist wards, with few highly trained nursing staff, intense medical interventions and control, plus a transient skilled agency nursing staff.

The highly specialised units led to students having a low profile and status, staying on one ward for short periods, and developing very short term relationships. Obviously such environments are very interesting to study to assess how students and even trained nursing staff develop and manage relationships. For example, both Melia's (1980) and Smith's (1992) studies were done in such environments which are usually a feature of large (medical)

64

teaching hospitals. However, the hospital and S.O. N. (1) I chose was typical of middle sized district hospitals with a mixture of few highly technical medical specialisms and standard acute services. I believed this standard hospital and College setting allowed social/ working boundaries to be more visible, and would hence make it easier to identify the properties of the relationships themselves. In choosing the small S.O. N.(1) I had worked in for two years I believe I was following Corsaro's (1980) recommendation for 'prior ethnography' of participant observer (in the native role):

> to provide a baseline of cultural accommodation and informational orientation that will be invaluable in increasing both the effectiveness and the efficiency of the formal work. (Corsaro 1980, p.9)

This choice also shows my bias to 'dance' between the Martian stance and the convert stance (Davis 1973), that is, trying to 'see' what I knew with 'new eyes', or to be:

> anthropologically strange, in an effort to make explicit the assumptions he or she takes for granted as a culture member. (Hammersley and Atkinson, 1983, p.8)

In line with Lofland and Lofland's, (1984, p.16) recommendation, I maintained a distance in observational work (the Martian view) by not getting into uniform and doing the work of nursing. As I was already a convert to the social setting from my previous work experience I had a reasonable access to understanding.

By the time I went into the fieldwork nearly three years had elapsed since I had left that School so I was less known to many people, which meant I had no personal work agenda which might have interfered with my role as researcher.

Most of the tutors I knew of old were still there, and some of the senior students I had known in their first few months of training were now preparing for final examinations. Most of the other students were unknown to me. This combination of being known by enough people but not part of the present day life of the school was a distinct advantage. It "broke the ice", so to speak, as tutors and senior students were able to vouch for my good intentions based on our previous working relationship. Yet, I was also seen as new and independent by the newer students and many of the ward staff whom I did not know.

The ward working context

An important social context in which interpersonal relating occurs is in the hospital wards where nurses work alongside other nurses and allied professions

65

in a multi-disciplinary team.

For this study, the hospital was a large district hospital servicing an urban population on the periphery of the capital city. The patient group spanned the whole range of social groups with an even mix of the very young, the very old, professional and working classes alike. The hospital provided the usual services to an urban area which included a large busy accident and emergency department. The hospital staff worked closely with a large community and psychiatric service where student nurses were allocated for short observational and some practical experience. The management team of the hospital was dominated by senior medical and nursing staff. The nurses had moved up the career ladder from clinical nursing to become clinical nursing officers under a Director of Nursing Service, who was also a trained nurse. This is significant for this research in that throughout most of the field work, while most hospitals in and around the country were grappling with the implications of the White Paper 'Working for Patients' (HMSO 1989) the purchaser and provider structure, this hospital seemed to allow new government policies to be implemented elsewhere before making changes itself. At ward level this strategy for managing change allowed for a relatively stable working atmosphere.

The ward nursing team generally consisted of the ward manager, (mostly ward sisters in this hospital) one senior staff nurse, as the ward manager's deputy, two junior staff nurses, or enrolled nurses, and three to five student nurses, ranging from post-registration students and first to third year students. (all training for Part 1 of the United Kingdom Central Council 1985 (UKCC)). The Project 2000 students were to follow, commencing training in late 1991 and only gaining significant ward experience in this hospital by late 1993. These students therefore, formed only a small but important part of this study through observation of their Interpersonal Skills Training and studying their evaluations of groupwork.

Most of the hospital wards were considered suitable for the allocation of students through a formal assessment by senior nurse educators in the College of Nursing and the Senior Nursing officers (senior clinical nurses in the hospital). The purpose of allocating students to wards for specified periods was to give them supervised educative experiences of nursing, where integration of the theory and practice of nursing would be expected to be seen to merge.

A mentorship system was in operation on the wards to supervise students during their experience. There is no mention of the role and function of the mentor in the curriculum document, (S.O.N.(1) 1989) and apart from the obligation to provide a verbal and written intermediate and final ward report, the quality of mentorship and the nature of the role was left to the individual staff nurse's or ward sister's preference. Details of progress in the clinical areas were recorded using the S.O.N.(1) progress report forms. Student nurses were allocated to different wards for periods of four weeks (in very specialised areas) to sixteen weeks in the more general areas such as general surgery, medicine and care of the elderly wards.

The main teaching occurred in the S.O.N (1). However the linking of the practical experience with theoretical knowledge was encouraged by planned weekly seminars on the wards. In fact the ward seminars were very erratic and depended on the number of staff on duty and whether the staff nurses liked teaching.

The educational working context

Relationships within nurse education developed with tutors and students engaged in the curriculum content, and where the operations involved in teaching and learning generated their own interpersonal processes. The tutor and student relationship needs to be placed in the context of a teaching / learning community in the School of Nursing. It seemed that the educational environment was the one place where it was possible to throw into relief the interpersonal dynamics which straddled the learning needs of nurses as individuals and the need for the profession to supply people who can do the job of nursing. It is in the School of Nursing that the tension is held between the government's promise to provide an effective and efficient nursing service and the education, personal and professional, of those who chose to join the nursing ranks. How the School tutors managed these tensions and implemented their educational strategy in terms of their educational relationship with students and to some degree, with the ward staff is the subject of discussion in Chapters 4, 5 and 6.

The School of Nursing (1) was on the threshold of making changes during the life of this research and in fact the staff went through an amalgamation with another School of Nursing (2) to form one major College of Nursing (1). Further changes were pending from regional strategy plans but tutors had yet to hear the real plans and therefore were optimistic about remaining where they were for at least three years. However, during the time that most of the interviews were done the School of Nursing remained relatively stable, so it was possible to perceive how tutors and students would relate to each other and how they had access to each other even when the students were on the wards.

The curriculum in operation at the time of the research was initiated in 1986 and revised in 1989. This curriculum was the last before the Project 2000 Diploma course was initiated in the amalgamated College of Nursing (1). Therefore the study was carried out in a time of transition, both in terms of the curricula and the College structure.

The School of Nursing (1) I was involved with, trained nurses for Part 1 of the Professional Register, (English National Board (ENB) 1983), that is a 146 week training for first time entrants. They also offered a 79 week (conversion) course for those already on other parts of the Professional Register, for example nurses already trained in Mental Health, Mental Handicap and Paediatric Nursing, as well as a 111 week course for nurses on Part 2 of the Register (enrolled nurse register) to convert to Part 1 of the Professional Register. By the end of the fieldwork this school was preparing to receive Project 2000-Diploma in Nursing students, from the other educational site and prepare them for observation work on the wards as part of their Common Foundation Course.

Formal access

Formal access to the School of Nursing (1) was granted to me by the Principal of the College following a written application. The Vice-Principal provided guidance and gave permission for contact with the tutors and students. A tutor's office was made available for interviews and internal posting facilities obtained to facilitate communication between the students on the wards and the S.O. N.(1) and myself. Complete freedom was given to me to approach any tutor or student and all curriculum documents needed were to hand. This part of the negotiations took one month and went smoothly. I was not so fortunate with gaining access to the wards as my initial correspondence was apparently mislaid. I wrote letters to the Clinical Nurse Managers of the two General Hospitals linked to the new College of Nursing and eventually succeeded in gaining the access needed. The procedure took many months and I decided to start my data collection with intensive interviews away from the wards and only use ward observations to see if I could recognise interpersonal relationship issues as described by nurses in the interviews.

For the ward observation I wanted wards where the students were allocated fora reasonable length of time; from ten to sixteen weeks. My reasons can be summed up with Melia's comment that nurses need:

> ..get to know the ward routine, know how Sister (and the other staff) likes things done...which takes about two weeks before you can settle down to nursing your patients and feeling part of the ward team. (Melia, 1987, p105)

Nurses on the three wards identified were given a letter of introduction which had a response slip attached for staff to sign by way of voluntarily inviting me into their wards for observational work. I was concerned that my entry be seen to be negotiated, so I used the return of the response slip as an indication of people's willingness to be observed and approached during observations. None of the ward staff availed themselves of pre-observational discussions which I offered and in fact most did not use the internal mail to post their responses back to me, but rather gave them to me when I arrived on the wards for my observations. The ward observations will be discussed later in this chapter.

Gaining access to participants

Davis (1986) described it well when she separated the process of gaining formal research entry with authority figures of the institution (who are not going to be the research respondents) and negotiating access to potential research respondents. Gaining access to the latter is to ask respondents to share their perceptions, their feelings and their interpersonal relationships with you as an unknown researcher. Building up a rapport which would enable people to want to share their inner world with you takes time and sensitive interpersonal dialogue. People need to see you as a 'trustworthy person and also credible as a researcher' if they are going to give you their time and tell you their story. (Lofland & Lofland 1984, p.25) Therefore I presented myself to my former colleagues as just that and as a student myself. Although I was no longer working in the Health Service, I was still accepted by them as a nurse tutor. They also knew of my interest in personal and interpersonal skills development and were very supportive of my study. As agreed with the Senior Tutor, I sent out letters of invitation to all the tutors (12 in total) and to most of the students in the S.O.N.(1) (110 in number) I wanted to interview student nurses who were at least six months into their training on the assumption that it was more probable that they would have built up some relationships within their learning set, with their tutors, as well as have some experience of relationships on the wards. I received responses from 55 per cent of the tutors within a short space of time, most agreed to be interviewed, three asked for an informal chat before committing themselves, which was an option I had offered. Four out of the 110 students responded in the affirmative in the first instance. I decided that face to face contact and word of mouth was probably a better introduction to students. In my letter of introduction, I had wanted to be honest and spell out what the intentions of the interviews were, but this was necessarily ambiguous, as I did not have a formal research question and I did not want to pre-determine the content or outcome of the interview. However the letters acted as a forerunner to my later contacts, as over the period of the study students did remember receiving the letter, but for various reasons, of which the pressure of time seemed the most pressing, they did not respond. Students and even staff nurses seeing me in the S.O.N.(1) and on the wards and hearing my request to observe them at work expressed curiosity at what I was doing and approached me. Once contact was made most people readily volunteered to be interviewed. Over the next nine months, through a snowball effect, I gradually completed the first round of interviews I needed.

Sampling

The form of sampling I used was a purposeful 'intensity' sampling (Patton 1990, pp.171-172) meeting the criteria of interpersonal relationships at their most usual working level, that is, student to student, tutor to student and student to junior trained ward staff. Senior tutors, ward managers (ward sisters) and other professional groups within the general hospital and college were not included as the relationship distance was potentially too wide and complicated by hierarchical and other organisational dimensions to be useful.
The importance of staying with "those cases that manifest sufficient intensity to illuminate the nature of success or failure" (Patton. op. cit.) of the phenomenon guided the sampling for this study. This purposeful sampling became more theory-based during the latter stages of the research as part of theoretical sampling (Patton 1990, pp.182-183), (see Chapter 2, Stage 5). The sample was not intended to be representative of all the tutors, students and junior trained staff, but rather an indepth focus on a small sample to elicit the social and psychological processes fuelling interpersonal relationships. (See Gregory 1994 for a more technical breakdown of participant and theoretical sampling.)

In this research, theoretical saturation of new concepts occurred with analysis of approximately 20 interview transcripts. The same descriptive phases, critical incidents and explanations and interpretations were offered by the interviewees speaking of the same or similar situations and across different situations (between the ward and the S.O.N.(1) and (2) and between different wards and different grades of nursing staff) pertaining to the interpersonal relationship dimension under study. At this point I ceased interviewing to collect new data, yet carried on discussing the findings with whoever cared to listen within the research field and continued to visit the wards and College of Nursing (1) informally to keep immersed in the research environment. This ongoing dialogue with interested parties helped me to constantly clarify ideas and refine emerging theory. The process of testing out emerging categories in this research took the form of:

1   Re-visiting some participants for further intensive interviews to develop content from the first cluster of interviews and to share my interpretation with them for clarification and verification

2   Sharing with my research support group the raw data and my coding techniques, critically assessing my efforts and skills to do constant comparative analysis, identify emerging categories and final conclusions. Checking that emerging hypotheses were grounded in the raw data.

3   Peer debriefing. (advocated by Lincoln and Guba 1985: 308 for researcher credibility).   This was done by an intensive prolonged interview between myself and a gestalt therapist in a peer relationship with me.   The purpose was to rattle and shake me on any implicit assumptions and biases I held that I might be imposing on the data (play devil's advocate).   This process also helped me to clarify my interpretations and to explore my findings from the perspectives of nursing culture and the Health Service organisation.   My research support group also played an important devil's advocate role in this respect.

4   Observing similar educational groupwork sessions with up to 16 student nurses in the groups (four 2 hour sessions) and of trained nursing staff doing specialist training (two 2 hour sessions) in two different Colleges of Nursing to look for incidents of the emerging concepts.   Seeking evaluations of experiential groupwork from the students and tutors of these groups for theoretical sampling .

5   Discussing the interpretation of my research with peer professionals on teacher training courses, again for confirmation of fit and relevance to their work relationships with students and the issues surrounding educational groupwork.

6   Submitting first level analysis and the developing theory of this research to a small number of interviewees to check if the emerging theory 'fitted' and 'worked' as defined in Chapter 2. (Stage 1)

Practical procedures surrounding intensive interviews

The intensive (focused conversation) interview technique was selected to engage participants in discussing issues addressing their interpersonal relationships with other nurses and nurse teachers at work both on the wards and in the S.O.N. (1).   This involved talking about their immediate work situation and retrospectively their relationships since they had entered the nursing profession.

Intensive interviewing is believed to be an effective way of helping interviewer and participant view each other as peers (after Lincoln & Guba 1985: 270), and therefore more likely to be comfortable talking to each other. The aim is to develop a quality of relating which is open and which respects the participant's unique and idiosyncratic viewpoint.   According to Lincoln and Guba (op cit: 270) this disposition with participants is necessary as it is they who hold both the questions and the answers about relationships within their social environment and they keep control of how much they share with the interviewer. Hence the informal dialogue was as much directed by what the participants believed to be important aspects of nursing and relationships as it was by my interest in nurse-nurse relationships per se.

The intensive interviews were conducted mainly in the S.O.N (1) where I had been offered an office. Other participants were interviewed in patients interview rooms within the wards where they worked, and one student was interviewed twice in her home as that was the most convenient venue for her. It was negotiated in advance that all interviews would be tape recorded, and this did not seem to pose a problem for participants. Informal discussions on the ward, over coffee in the Schools of Nursing, and during discussions of the research with student groups outside the research site (for the purpose of triangulation) were written up as fieldnotes either at the time or very shortly afterwards.

The method of interviewing was based on a facilitative encounter. Heron's (1989b and 1990) Six Category Intervention Analysis model was intentionally used with particular emphasis on catalytic, supportive and `gentle' confrontative interventions. In the questioning technique a process of laddering was used, moving from peripheral or surface concerns to more core feelings,values, beliefs and problems. The process moved from description, reflection to critical reflection with each new concept under discussion, similar to Hammersley and Atkinson's (1983, p.113) "reflexive interviewing." In this way, it was possible to obtain behavioural and other concrete characteristics of concepts (description); move to the conceptual meaning and labels given to experience by the participants, (reflection) onto uncovering the underlying assumptions about the content, context, theorising and decisions they made about their relationships (critical reflection) (after Tosey 1993). I found that this approach had the effect of confronting people's implicit assumptions and causing them to question why they do what they do. This consequence of an intensive research process was also found by Sims (1981, p.373) which he described as participants moving from `ethogeny to endogeny'. Such a method of interviewing facilitates insights into aspects of a person's values and behaviour which they may not have been aware of and may not feel comfortable with. It may also highlight to them the state of their relationships at work which may be unsettling for them. I encountered some of these issues with different participants at interview, which supported Wilde's (1992) experience of "breaking the rules" when participants discussed emotionally charged situations. In anticipation of participants becoming unsettled during or after the interviews I finished each interview with gradually bringing the person to a comfortable level of social awareness and offering them follow-up counselling or discussion as necessary. My training as a one-to-one and group facilitator enabled me to offer ongoing support as required. Each participant was given my home address, and work and home telephone number; however, none of the participants took up the invitation.

The first few minutes of each interview were concerned with checking their signed consent as evidence of the voluntary nature of the interview and giving them more information about myself if it was requested. Confidentiality was an important issue, although some said they were comfortable for others to know who they were and how they felt. However on invitation, all participants chose a code by which they would be referred to in the transcripts and any other field-notes I would make. Once all questions were answered the participants were again given the opportunity to decide to carry on to the interview. In the first round of interviews the first and only predetermined questions asked were:

1   How long have you been in nursing?
2   What does nursing mean to you?

The interview then unfolded with my questions arising out of the data as offered. The content moved between their nursing duties, their relationships with other nurses in the wards and in the S.O.N. (1). Nurses seemed to gravitate easily to talking about the nurse-patient relationship and had more difficulty staying with their personal and interpersonal relationship with other nurses. In retrospect I noticed that to some degree I directed the focus of attention to the educational opportunities which might address the interpersonal issues in the form of interpersonal training and how this influenced their relationships with each other as nurses. Hammersley & Atkinson (1983, pp.113-114) suggest that such directing of interview content is important "to keep the research focus". All raw data from the first round of intensive interviews were transcribed, and in subsequent interviews the salient features were also transcribed. All conversational notes, discussions and observational data were added to the growing database at the appropriate level of analysis. An example of first level data analysis through to tentative development of theoretical categories is offered as Appendix B. The nature of the research was such that I could only interview one or two participants and then I needed to sort raw data into codes and develop tentative categories from the raw data before interviewing more participants; to do otherwise would have made it difficult and inappropriate to do constant comparative analyses, to build on ideas and possible categories already emerging and to do theoretical sampling. Thus six months were spent slowly transcribing data and interviewing at irregular intervals.

After this initial analysis of data I began to look again at the nursing, nurse education and social/ medical psychological literature to check if my findings linked with concepts and theories already available. Those findings will be discussed in their fully developed form in Chapters 4, 5 and 6. As a result of the analysis at that time I was particularly keen to interview more students and trained staff . In the meantime, I gave participants already interviewed copies of their transcribed interviews and arranged to re-interview some of them. I wanted to get written comments from them about my tentative interpretations of the issues surrounding interpersonal relationships between nurses. This was done to check out some of the concepts and categories that were emerging to ascertain that I was representing their views accurately and to explore in more depth the emerging categories.

After 18 months of individual intensive interviews and many informal discussions, plus the results of the observations, I concluded that I was working through the same cycles of events in terms of people's stories, my own perceptions and evidence gathered from the research site and outside it through theoretical sampling. I decided to take it that the categories were fully saturated for the salient features I had focused on. I had hoped to glean more from the interpersonal skills training in the S.O.N.(1) as both tutors and students spoke to me as though the interpersonal skills strand of the curriculum was in action. Even in the analyses it seemed present, yet this category seemed weakly grounded in any concrete examples, that is, I could not define the properties well in descriptive terms, even though they were embedded in intellectual discourse about `what should happen'. I concluded that this weakness in grounding the concepts in practice meant that nurses were not training specifically in interpersonal skills, regardless of the verbatim data. On return to the research site I asked each of the tutors:

> Over the past few years, who in the School has been teaching the interpersonal skills strand of the curriculum?

The response was

> Nobody specifically, some of us talk about it to our students, but none of us feel qualified to teach it.

This confirmed what I was finding in the data and highlighted a blind spot I had as a researcher. I was quiet certain that interpersonal skills training was an active part of the curriculum and therefore I had not asked enough probing questions about what and how it was taught. My perceptions were also (mis)informed by the ease with which students and trained staff explored the link between interpersonal issues on the wards and the interpersonal skills training in the School, yet, I had not seen, on first analysis that many of the responses were in the imperative rather than the actual. To combat this problem, I re-opened my exploration of interpersonal skills training by interviewing a tutor designated to do this in the other School of Nursing (2) which made up the newly formed amalgamated College of Nursing. These discussions are integrated into the findings discussed in Chapters 4 and 5. I observed this tutor teaching interpersonal skills on two separate occasions and spoke to some of her students. With their permission I have included some of their evaluations of learning interpersonal skills in their stable group.

Discussion on ward observation can be found Gregory (1994). The last section of this Chapter will be an overview of the sorting and re-sorting of data into theoretical categories: stating which data stayed in the melting pot as ingredients for further analysis and which data were put aside and why.

Initial sorting of data into codes and categories

The initial sorting of data proved more difficult than I had imagined, partly because I thought it should be a complicated process so made it so, and partly because it was complicated in ways I did not yet know. Transcribing every word, underlining every sentence which might be significant (yet not knowing what was significant in the early stages) and most importantly not being rigorous enough in eliminating all data which were not related to the unit of analysis meant that initial data accumulated faster than was manageable. It was inappropriate to impose such rigour in the early stages, nonetheless the consequences were that I felt swamped by the data. All data `bits' (sentences illustrating a concept) were typed separately, photocopied, the originals filed and the copies pasted together on A4 pages according to the relational clusters and categories assigned to them. However these remained at a descriptive rather than a conceptual level, so there was a need to shift to another level of labelling phenomena (see Chapter 2, Stage 1.).

A further sorting was done to open up the data more into ascriptive categories as a way of managing the data by groupings, such as tutor-tutor relationship, tutor-student relationship, student-student, student-trained staff and nurse-patient relationships. This sorting illustrated who talked to whom and in what place as much as what they said and was done to identify the properties and dimensions of a category (Chapter 2, Stages 2 and 3). The codings clustered in the following way with raw data `bits' given to illustrate each coding.

Figure 3.1 Ascriptive categories

Descriptive coding:	Verbatim accounts:
1) Interpersonal skills:	"You need to be aware of how you feel about situations before you have to deal with them with another person, another party." (Student)
2) Educational Groupwork:	"Nurses are afraid they will be put down by other nurses, so they avoid giving feedback or validation, so that it is not given to them in return." (Tutor)
3) Hiding behind the Uniform:	"You hide behind the uniform, when I talk to patients, I behave differently. I have seen nurses do that. Go from being shy in social situation, to being confident to asking complete strangers (patients) the most personal details." (Tutor)
4) Nurse Hierarchical Relationships:	"Demanding patients should only be confronted by the Sister or Doctor or Staff Nurse. Students should complain to trained staff if a patient is being unreasonable. They can say, "You are not the only patient on the ward." (Student)
5) Peer-Peer Relationship, The non-Trusting Environment:	"People working together as peers are not being open and sharing what they feel about things, about what they see as wrong, it's avoiding conflict."
6) Teamwork on the Ward:	"Generally nurses working on the ward get on, they have to, or else there won't be unity and the nursing will fall apart." (Student)

Descriptive coding:	Verbatim accounts:
7) Student nurse-Tutor relationship:	"Even in School, we are too bound up in the curriculum content to give students time to talk about their feelings and attitudes." (Tutor)
8) What Nursing is:	"Nursing is an individual thing, you can't nurse two people in the same way, and if students find that out, and I have helped them, that's important, because it would be lasting and will change their attitude to patients." (Student)
9) Nurses' Emotional / Skills Needs:	"There is a double bind; nurses need to have some practical / conceptual understanding of nursing to understand the educational processes, yet the educational approach is to prepare them to nurse." (Tutor)
10) No Time to Care:	"Nurses used to be busier, with lots of non-nursing duties, now all those have been taken away and still they seem to have less time to sit with patients, not all nurses, but most of them." (Tutor)

I held these crude categories for approximately twelve months, gradually building up different data `bits' in different sorting files and creating a picture of the recurring themes which were part of `being in College' and `being on the wards', in the vein of *constant comparative analysis* (Chapter 2, Stage 2 & 3). Through using the six "C's" to question the data, the coding moved from the descriptive to the conceptual, and from the concrete to the abstract. The method to do this is through theoretical memos which is an essential skill in theory generation. The more this developed the more I realised the logic and in theory the simplicity of the data analysis. What needed to happen was to "Hear the music behind the message" as in a therapeutic encounter, or in good communication skills generally. This process extracts the meaning from the data, rather than repeating the data using different words. Having that clarification I decided I was ready to "intuitively" feel for what people were saying to me, imagining them sitting with me in the interview. I listened to all the taped interviews again, read all the memos to date plus all the fieldnotes looking for process codes, dynamic codes of doing and being, thinking and feeling. From this the above categories were re-sorted to reflect more the sociopsychological processes which seemed to be going on. This essential shift to look for theoretical codes as opposed to descriptive codes facilitated the development of conceptual categories. This way of grounding theory from raw data through substantive coding, concept formation to theoretical categories was the strategy used in this research. The danger of staying descriptive rather than moving into discovery mode, that is to "the conceptualisation of an underlying social process at an abstract level" was well voiced by Becker (1993). I recognised that I was in that descriptive mode with much of the data for many months.

I was reluctant at this stage to put aside data which addressed the relationship between nurse and patient. I imagined that how nurses related to each other could affect how they responded to patients, and this was borne out at interview. Also from a utilitarian viewpoint, it seemed to give more justification for the study if it could be seen that nurses' relationship with each other did have an effect on their relationship with patients. So for another six months I carried on in the theoretical sampling to monitor this dimension of relationships on the wards.

The revised substantive codes clustered into 13 new "theoretical" categories illustrated below.

Figure 3.2 Initial theoretical categories

Theoretical categories:	Verbatim data:
1) Interpersonal relating with patients	`You can't demonstrate your nursing skills unless you actually communicate with people. get their permission to do nursing.' (Staff Nurse)
2) Being emotionally competent to help others	`I think nurses who stand up for their own rights and their patients rights are valuable'. (Tutor)
3) Having power and control over (other nurses)	`Nurses don't treat their own colleagues well when they become patients. I guess it's fear of doing something wrong and being found out and criticised.' (Tutor)

Theoretical categories (contd):	Verbatim data (contd):
4) Supporting each other (positive and negative examples)	`Need to recognise our attitudes, be self-aware, to be supportive of others (nurses)'. (Tutor) `Nurses are all going through their own stresses so they are unable to look at others, see their stress and help them'. (Student)
5) Caring in a clinical way	`With staff and supervising tutors, if you get your work done, they (the staff) will not notice that you are not being caring, but if you are caring, but equally efficient, they would recognise that'. (Student)
6) Working to hide caring: Using work to avoid personal contact	`I see a lot of nurses' coping strategies, on duty and off: the degree of avoidance, the unpopular patient, the patient whom they feel uncomfortable with. So patients don't get much attention, nurses chatter among themselves'. (Tutor)
7) Developing a personal power	`Relationships with colleagues, assertiveness might be useful if the teacher is good. But inner strength is more important, which is self acquired, not taught'. (Student)
8) Nursing as it should be: the "shoulds" and the "should nots"	`Junior nurses should not be given patient assessments to do, senior nurses should do this'. (Tutor)
9) Confronting interpersonal conflict (or potential conflict)	`Nurses are silent about poor standards of care. They are frightened of having their cards marked'. (Student)

Theoretical categories (contd):	Verbatim data (contd):
10) Appropriate professional behaviour; doing it right.	`Nurses have a professional aspect to their work. They also have personal aspects which might impinge on the profession'. (Student)
11) Learning by doing	Students have to learn how to relate therapeutically to patients by experiences on the ward. They may learn by mistakes, which is going to be a bit unfortunate for them and for the patients. This experience will give them automatic responses to actual situations (in crises)'. (Tutor)
12) Meeting students' needs:	`Each student has their own individuality and if you (tutor) can be part of them finding that out, it is important, because the effects will be lasting and will affect their attitudes, knowing their own potential as an individual'. (Tutor)
13) Educational groupwork	`Unprepared people (students) will not open up in large groups. People have problems with coping with emotions'. (Tutor)

The 13 categories were sorted and re-sorted to check for duplication at a process level and at a higher level of abstraction, that is, were the same processes being discussed under different labels. It was important that the categories be mutually exclusive and embrace all the elements of the concepts to which they referred. It was equally important not to push codes into categories they did not belong to. Such a process was time consuming with constant re-appraisal of the data. The need to separate what was explanation of the data as descriptive events and what was explanation of personal and interpersonal contact and behaviour, based on their purpose (goal/motive) for the individual, was a necessary shift to theoretical sense making. The aim was to offer explanation-by-understanding at a theoretical level to foster prediction and theory generation. (Chapter 2, combination of Stages 4-6).

True to form, aa recounted in much of the literature on grounded theory, (Corbin, 1986: 92) so much data had been collected that the research questions and I were almost submerged for many months in a sea of confusion. Stepping back from the data and creating stronger theoretical concepts to higher levels of abstraction finally allowed me to manage the complexity and volume of the data. To this end the categories were resorted to form process categories, focusing more on the dynamic process words or "gerund" at a higher level of abstraction. One result from this sorting was that it allowed for the exclusion of data which referred to the nurses' desired or real relationship with patients which was not the unit of analysis under study. Much of the interpersonal processes in relationship with peers and seniors were mirrored in relationships with patients so the essences of the link with patients was not lost. However, the study was in danger of over-extending its boundaries into clinical nursing, to the detriment of the educational and social boundaries among nurses themselves, so a cut off point was made. It was at this stage that the fenced-off area in figure 1.3 (see Chapter 1) had to be taken seriously.

The categories which were excluded from this study were collectively called: The Ethos of Caring, which combined three categories: Making Contact with Patients- Interpersonal Relating with Patients; Caring versus Work-too busy to care (quality of caring); Caring versus Work- using work to avoid personal contact (with patients). This also included some codes from the first sorting under the heading of: Hiding behind the Uniform. The remaining categories were explored in more detail (Chapter 2, Stage 6 and 7.) for linkages between concepts and sub-categories, using the six `C"s (Chapter 2, stage 1). Following this, hierarchical taxonomies were developed enabling the salient sub-categories and finally the core sociopsychological processes to be identified.

The socio-psychological processes identified were taken back into the research field and checked with participants. It was at this stage that most of the theoretical sampling was done. For many months I re-visited the field, spoke to students, staff nurses and tutors, took my findings to my research support group, peer debriefing and to nurse training groups, both students and trained staff. I followed Stages 8 and 9 (Chapter 2) as far as it was relevant for this study. For extreme comparisons, I used my own experience as a facilitator of a two year experiential group and a training group in which I was a student and a specialist nurse training group outside of the research field.

At this juncture, without any discussion, I will give a list of the main salient categories of how nurses worked and related to each other as found in this study. Appendix B illustrate the process in more detail using two interviews in particular as examples, and Chapters 4, 5 and 6 will discuss the research findings with verbatim accounts to support the theoretical categories. These main categories are: .

The core category, which is also a socio-psychological process:

Fearing to trust and feeling vulnerable (as processes) which became subsumed under the category: Fearing intimacy in the form of openness about self and honesty with others.

The main basic socio-psychological process as a strategy:
　　　With-holding self as a strategy for self-management

Auxiliary categories:
　　　Living the contradiction in education
　　　Learning about self
　　　Belonging in the learning set
　　　Conformity to try to belong to the ward team
　　　The professional shield
　　　Power and control

Some of these categories with their elements are shown diagrammatically in the discussion chapters to follow.

Conclusion

In this Chapter, my intention was to open up for scrutiny my understanding and application of grounded theory, so that its suitability for the proposed research could be judged by other researchers. The mix of intensive interviews, some non-participant observations and casual visits both in the School of Nursing (1) and (2) and on wards in the general hospital, informal dialogue with many nurses, studying documentations and sharing research findings with research participants and peers formed the necessary data triangulation to give predictive validity to the emerging theory.

The section on initial sorting of data into coded categories goes further forward in the research by showing the emerging categories without sufficient description and illumination of the analysis. This was done to give an overview of the findings. Appendix B goes further still in demonstrating the microanalysis of data from the first two interviews as these laid the foundation for further comparative analysis and theoretical sampling.

A critique of the research approach adopted for this research will form part of the final chapter.

PART TWO
Discussion of findings

4 The educational relationship

Introduction

Two of the main focuses of education can be described as: education which is in the business of imparting information and developing the student, providing the `educated with more and different ways to view their world' (Bevis 1989); and the relationship between the teacher and students, as Pittenger and Gooding (1971) believed. This Chapter takes the latter focus without dismissing the former. The relationship referred to here is how both tutors and students interact in a social, psychological and educational way with each other.

A reminder of the research questions is given to show how these were explored within the educational setting. The questions were:

1   What are your interpersonal relationships like, with each other as students, with tutors, with ward staff?

2   Personal and interpersonal skills training is part of nurse training. How might they raise personal and interpersonal relationship issues for you, both in the School of Nursing and on the wards?

Answers to these questions were sought by synthesising the data using the six `C's devised by Glaser (1978) and described in Chapter 2. The aim is to describe the research story in an abbreviated form and offer a diagram showing the core category and its relationship with other categories which are sub-categories to the main category. An analytical explanation will then be given of how the core category and subcategories were derived from the data and in what way the core category is a `basic sociopsychological process' (Strauss & Corbin 1990, pp.121-123) (see also Chapter 2). The core category identified is: With-holding self-as a strategy for self-management.

To give an overview of the emerging theory the main core categories and socio-psychological processess are presented in one figure (**Figure 4.1**) in advance of the discussion to highlight to the reader the range of concepts that will be discussed. However, as will be seen in Chapters 4 and 6 these core categories and basic socio-psychological processed emerged from the data. The preferred style of presentating the conclusions is through an inductive process with propositions following the analysis rather than preceding them and this stlye will be followed in this book.

Figure 4.1 Mapping the elements of the substantive theory of "Withholding self as a strategy for self management"

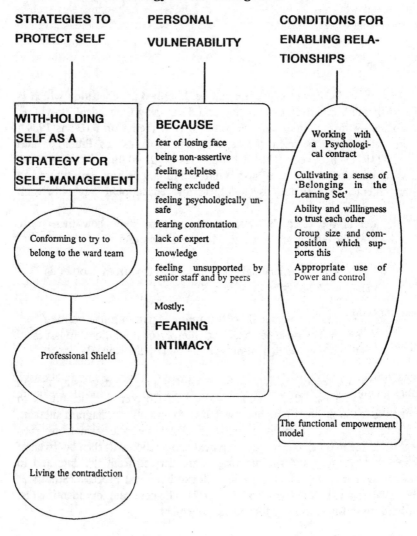

The core category: With-holding self as a strategy for self-management

The main story is reflected in the phenomenon I experienced which was one of 'not knowing what data were missing'. The participants in the study talked freely and willingly about their perceptions of interpersonal relationships within the School of Nursing and the hospital wards. In the tutors' accounts it was possible to believe that what was being said about interpersonal skills training was happening in reality, yet that turned out not to be the case. In the wards, student nurses and staff nurses talked of their working relationship, saying what was good and what was not so good. The general impression derived from all this data was that although the need for a positive interpersonal working environment for both nurses and patients was seen as important, this was an illusion, and another interpersonal dynamic, something not quite tangible, orchestrated how people really behaved. This was mirrored in the interviews, which although sometimes very probing, still had the sense of data falling through your fingers. Difficulties of definition of terms, whether they were being used on a social level or psychological level, and personal ownership or accountability for the interpersonal dynamics in existence seemed important characteristics which needed exploration. The illusion was even more difficult to define in the ward observations, where it manifested itself most potently in the 'disappearing nurses' when there was no 'real nursing' to be done (This will be discussed in Chapter 6). The illusion could later be identified as sociopsychological processes not known or in awareness at the start of the study, but which turned out to be, potentially, the driving force in interactions.

During the analysis of data I found myself asking; 'what's not being said while we are busy talking about this or that phenomenon?' What was not being said is summed up by the core category of with-holding as a method or strategy of psychological self management. Consulting Roget's Thesaurus (1962) on the word 'with-holding' other words were; hindrance, holding-in, bottling up, constraint, entrenchment, protectionism, as well as, to gag, to silence and so on. Such concepts are synonymous with many of the sub-categories in these chapters. The concept of with-holding self in interpersonal relating reflects a need to keep a distance from what is considered an intimacy (Appendix C), or an enabling or therapeutic relationship. An enabling or therapeutic relationship implies a contract between helper and helped which is a therapeutic encounter in the form of a journey that both will take with the intention of improving a life situation for one or both in the relationship. Such is the nature of empathy as defined by Rogers (1967) (see Chapter 1). Figure 4.1. illustrates the core category and the main sub-categories in relationship to with-holding.

Figure 4.2 With-holding self as a strategy for self-management (1)

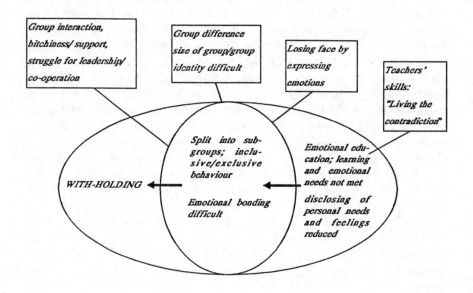

This chapter will proceed with opening up the sub-categories to identify in what way they relate to the core category of With-holding.

`Living the contradiction' in education

As stated in the introduction, the quest was to identify what might be some of the underlying issues linked with interactive interpersonal skills training. This category, `Living the contradiction' in education is a major sub-category linked with this quest as illustrated by the following:

> Although we say we are student centred, it's not really so, as most teachers would feel guilty about how much of the curriculum they have to cover. (Tutor)

> Even in School we are too bound up in the curriculum to give students time to talk about their feelings and attitudes. (another Tutor)

This highlights the juggling act which teachers perceived they were involved in between teaching a patient-centred curriculum and a student-centred educational process. I am associating student-centred learning with teachers taking account of students learning needs; emotional, intellectual, behavioural and spiritual which are aspects of the educated person (Heron 1974) as described in Chapter 1. as well as facilitating students to cultivate creative, dynamic modes of approaching patient care. (Bevis 1989) It is interesting to note that tutors said that they would feel guilty if they spent time negotiating educational needs with learners beyond imparting clinical and technical knowledge. By clinical I mean patient focused medical treatment and nursing care. It would seem that the clinical content dictated the teaching, rather than the learning and experiences students brought to the School of Nursing which might need expression and critical reflection. The seeming obligation for teachers to 'deliver the whole curriculum content' (Rolfe 1993, pp.149-154), before students can be assessed does place the emphasis heavily on the teacher to fulfil this professional obligation. This does not fit with the model of self-directed learning advocated by Knowles (1978, p.54) but rather the model of dependence, reminiscent of pedagogy, which is contrary to the stated educational philosophy of the School of Nursing (see Chapter 1). Where it does link is with the whole debate about educational power. For example, Lancaster (1972), Gott (1982), Rolfe (1993) found that nurse teachers believed that they should control learning, and that they had a professional responsibility to ensure that the curriculum was 'covered'. In this study, it was as though tutors felt guilty about spending teaching time focusing on students' needs, that if students failed examinations, and the tutor has not covered the subject 'properly' then it was the tutors' fault. Another possibility could be that the tutors' lack of ability or inclination to create opportunities for students to discuss their experiences and feelings was at the heart of how they prioritised curriculum content. This will be discussed more fully in next section; Learning about self. For now, here is an example of where student centred teaching seemed to work:

> I allow myself to get side tracked onto issues the students want to explore, and they tell me it's ok, it's what they want.

The same tutor:

Students will always learn what they need to learn to pass exams, and they learn this knowledge on the wards. In the school we should concentrate on attitudes which might not be picked up elsewhere.

For this tutor, exploring attitudes, (the individual's predisposition to think, feel and act in particular ways, depending on the person's values) through interactive discussion was part of personal development, a teaching strategy which ward nursing staff may not want to or be able to address. This tutor's statements showed her belief in the students' ability to be self-directed in pursuing their educational needs as and where appropriate which she then reflected in her teaching.

The difference between the educational task and educational process needs to be clarified. According to Heron, (1993, p.113) the educational task focuses on goals, teaching programme, teaching methods and giving conceptual understanding to experience, whereas the educational process mainly deals with feelings, confrontation and valuing within and between individuals. Although the process is powerfully influenced by the task, it can also be described separately. Others, for example, Bruner (1960), Stenhouse (1975), and Bevis (1989) concur with the definition above. They also put the main emphasis in valuing the learning process and learning experience, rather than with specific achievement outcomes, which is exemplified by Steinaker & Bell's (1979) taxonomy of experiential objectives. Even within the teaching methods referred to by Heron above under tasks, the teaching style can be either content focused or process focused (Gibbs 1992). Managing the educational process, and in fact, actively encouraging it to emerge through interactive and experiential teaching methods, (see Chapter 1) is an important dimension in personal development and interpersonal skills training. Jaques makes this point when he says:

> Where emphasis is placed on process learning and interaction in small groupwork there does appear to be a growth in student commitment... (to learning) (Jaques, 1991, p.20)

The 'juggling' between the delivery of a patient-centred curriculum content and the educational processes directed towards facilitating personal qualities (Burnard & Morrison (1989) can be mapped as in Figure 4.2.

Figure 4.3 Patient-centred curriculum and student-centred educational processes

CURRICULUM CONTENT	EDUCATIONAL PROCESSES
Focusing on theoretical and clinical knowledge	attitudes and values emerge here
assessed work from above	not assessed
students judged on these results	neither student nor tutors
tutors judged on these results	judged on these attributes

Figure 4.2 corresponds to the differences between the two educations as described by Jarvis (1986) and also recognised within nurse education by Gijbels. (1993) Beattie (1987) advocated a fourfold curriculum to embrace the classical with the romantic curricula at an ideological level with the product of education and educational processes at a practical level as a way of balancing what to others is an impossible merger. (Jarvis 1986)

It seems likely that tutors are 'uncomfortably' working across the two curricular models, that is 'education from above (versus) education of equals'. (Jarvis 1986, pp.465-469) Education from above fits the traditional notion of education, which is, the 'moulding of the person' to fit the system into which they are being absorbed, in this case, into nursing. The education of equals, on the other hand, puts the educational needs of the individual first, and personal learning as the pivot on which curriculum content is negotiated and directed. As Rolfe (1993) says, this does not fit the ongoing assessment and examination procedures for entry into the nursing profession (English National Board (ENB) 1990) so would not be given a high priority, if given any priority at all. This confirms the finding in this research when, in theoretical sampling, I approached some tutors in a different College of Nursing, whose main teaching involvement was the interpersonal skills training. I shared with them my tentative interpretations of tutors in the research School of Nursing (S.O.N. (1)) prioritising curriculum content to match examination requirements rather than what they thought students really needed. I asked these 'new' tutors how they thought their work was accepted by students and what value it was given within the College of Nursing. Their reply was surprising. The tutors said they felt the Cinderella team of the College with students giving low priority to attendance at their workshops and disregarding their reflective journals, yet the tutors empathised with the students' position. It was their empathy which surprised me. When I asked why they felt such empathy, the response was simple:

> They don't get assessed on the interpersonal skills module. They get assessed on everything else, so they put interpersonal skills knowledge and practice to the end of their learning needs. We don't blame them either, so we take what we can and do what we can with the students. (Tutors)

I suggested to one of the tutors, that such a belief from the tutorial team, that it is all right (understandable) for students to put interpersonal skills training at the end of their list of priorities could affect how students viewed the importance of this subject as part of their nurse training. The tutor agreed and thought that the effect was a negative one, but reiterated that such was the reality in nurse education.

So even those tutors whose main work was to develop the personal and professional qualities in nurses seemed to believe that in the final analysis, such personal qualities came second to clinical knowledge and skills. The friction seems to be a schism between individual tutors' values which seemed to agree with the stated intentions within the curriculum documents on the one hand; on student centred learning, and tutors' behaviour on the other. And the sense of guilt could be the discomfort with `living the contradiction'. Living the incongruence between the espoused practice, which is, in the main, the education of equal and the actual practice, which is education from above. The rationalisation for this sociopsychological process of `living the contradiction' is that although tutors want nurses to learn how to be person-centred, they cannot demonstrate this in educational outcomes. It would seem that the end justifies the means, that is, passing assessments drives what and how curriculum content is covered and tutors feel a need to accept this state of affairs. This hypothesis corresponds with Rolfe's (1993, p.149) assessment of what he termed `the constraints of the nursing professional curriculum'. However, I believe the constraints are self-imposed by virtue of trying to integrate two different beliefs about the nature of the person, and what constitutes educational processes into a curricular model. Such an integration creates educational programmes in conflict between personal learning processes and achievement outcomes.

With the core category of `With-holding self-as a strategy for self-management' identified as a basic sociopsychological process, that is, a problem which nurses are trying to manage in the educational context, the question is, in what way is `Living the contradiction' a property (sub-category) of the core category. The answer lies in the tension between the educational task and educational processes. It will be seen throughout the section on `Learning about self' which will follow, that the students see the philosophical confusion; they experience the contradiction between learning clinical knowledge, and learning how to manage their personal and interpersonal skills. They know that clinical knowledge, theoretical and practical, is all that is assessed and rewarded, so with-hold self from whole-heartedly engaging in the educational processes which they experience as most vulnerable, and without obvious educational rewards, that is, experiential ways of working in interpersonal skills training.

If the investment of time in the College is in the clinical education of student nurses, the question arises as to what might be happening to the emotional education within the espoused holistic educational philosophy? This will be covered in the next section. However, I believe one can draw some tentative hypotheses from the above category, that is; that tutors exercise control over what part of the curriculum gets greater emphasis, clinical knowledge or personal and interpersonal development; that the summative assessments influence prioritisation of the curriculum content, sometimes against the tutors' better judgement; and possibly, that tutors decide the teaching styles they use depending on their biases and abilities both in teaching methods and content expertise. The relational link, in terms of axial coding between 'Living the contradiction' and 'With-holding' within the paradigm model (Strauss & Corbin 1990, p.99) is that 'Living the contradiction' is the context in which students learn of the tutors' ability to activate the curricular philosophy. The consequence of tutors ambiguity trying to move between the two curriculum models creates confusion and with-holding. As Jarvis said:

A significant feature of this analysis (of the two educations) is that education cannot be neutral, it is one or the other... possibly in the course of teaching and learning, some teachers may switch from one to another, although they may not be consciously aware of the process through which they are going. (Jarvis 1986: 467)

Argyris (1964) offered a theory which has some bearing here on how student nurses could have picked up the psychological messages of ideal versus real educational and nursing practice when he identified the 'espoused theory' and 'theory-in-use'. This model shows the incongruence which occurs between what people say they do (in terms of philosophy and ideal intentions) and what actually happens. Argyris maintains that people hold these two theories implicitly, the theory in use being the one that guides them in everyday action, and the espoused theory, the one they say they believe in. These two theories may or may not be compatible, indeed the individual or group may not perceive the discrepancy between the two theories, as they will use strategies to restrict outcome which supports their theory-in-use, which Argyris terms single loop learning.

Learning about self

This section will develop the concepts and categories relating to facilitating learning about self as a major sub-category of 'With-holding self as a strategy for self-management'. Using the six 'C' model (Chapter 2) this category is the psychosocial and intrapsychic context in which both the behaviour of with-holding and the concepts of 'belonging to' occur. How the category 'Learning about self' emerged will be demonstrated by the distillation of data into properties of the category which showed up as conditions and strategies of the core processes addressing the education of the person within the professional context.

The sub-categories are: emotional education; belonging in the learning set; trusting self and others as an educative process; mutual feedback and peer support; and disclosing self to others.

The section will finish with a diagrammatic presentation of core categories and suggested basic psychosocial processes motivating the interpersonal relationships within the educational institution, particularly through the learning processes. Although the section is divided into sub-sections to present the data more clearly, yet the inter-relationship between all the concepts and categories should be held in the mind of the reader, as they are held in the working dynamic for participants.

Emotional education

During interviews the topic of emotional needs and emotional competence (see Chapter 1.) was raised in the context of how nurses managed their interpersonal relations both in the School of Nursing and on the hospital wards. Many tutors saw the expression of feelings and attitudes as important educational requirements. For example:

> If I have a group of students I share my feelings and thoughts and they do the same, and about how they feel bad on the ward, and they say how they would like it to be. (Tutor).

In a follow up interview I asked a Tutor what her definition of feelings / emotions was to which she replied:

> Emotions ..are feelings... it comes from within, the feeling that you have within, whether it's being upset and crying or being happy,..or something along those lines. I find it very difficult to describe.

And a student:

Emotions are all those things that turn around inside you, particularly when things are not going right.

Both definitions of emotions are similar and correspond with Heron's (1992) definition (see Chapter 1).

Kagan (1985) was quite emphatic when she said that the place of emotions in teaching interpersonal skills training required a special relationship between teachers and students. In this study, exploring what tutors and students thought of each other led to some diverse comments. For example, most tutors said that they recognised the need to see the student as a person with rights and not solely as a provider of patients' needs. How these sentiments were reflected in practice was explored in some of the interviews. Did student nurses feel cared for in a manner that reflects the definition of an enabling relationship as defined by Rogers (1967) (see endnote 2 in Chapter 1). One student discussing how she was treated on the ward regarding ageism said:

> Oh, yes. But mind you I feel like that with the tutors anyway. I feel a lot that they speak down, they don't mean to, I mean they are used to speaking to.., I suppose, on the whole.., to younger- but then, why really. I don't think anyone should speak down to anyone.

She went on to say that some tutors are informal and comfortable to be with, that they can have good discussions, and a laugh which she liked:

> I do get support from my tutor. When we had two exams on top of each other, he offered to help. I said, "Well, I wouldn't mind a chat about it" and he said "Yeah, no problem, when it's convenient for you." He is not one of those people who will badger you all the time- he is always there... and I suppose he is our advocate as well... he sticks up for us on the wards about our continuous assessments. (Student)

This student was referring to the one-to-one relationship with her tutor which she saw as facilitative. Such facilitative relationship with tutors was confirmed by many students. It was the relationship in the classroom that seems to be at variance with the facilitative relationship advocated. As the student, Andy, said:

> Everybody keeps it *(their problems)* to themselves. Like a couple of lassies who started, really homesick, they asked the tutor if they could have a word, but the tutor did nothing...Like there is no team spirit.... The teacher is in the group to get team spirit going, but nothing ever

happens. There is little respect for most teachers as they can't keep control.

Andy is not advocating power sharing in terms of equal responsibility in maintaining order in the educational process, but rather expects the teacher to impose discipline.

Some contradictions appeared between some tutors' perceptions of their ability to create a good learning relationship which would encourage sharing of feelings and attitudes and some students' perceptions that the relationship was not facilitative, that the power position of the tutors was a hindrance to openness in the group, and that the skills of the tutors make a difference to how secure and trusting students felt. (This will be discussed further in the section discussing the category 'Trusting self and others' later in this chapter).

In one interview with a tutor, we had been talking about student distress on the wards and I asked:

> JG: So how do you think students manage otherwise, if they don't actually overtly show they are not managing? (their emotions following experiencing a traumatic event such as a death or a resuscitation)

She replied:

> Tutor: Sometimes the students come to the school for support, but they are often too anxious, pathologically sometimes. So when they are in school I recognise that they are unhappy and ask them what is wrong. It usually surprises them that you have noticed their unhappiness.

(By pathological, this tutor meant when the students were very depressed with a sense of not wanting to carry on nursing).

> JG: Because, somehow they have... got the notion that on the ward they will really have to break down or overtly ask for help before it is given?

> Tutor: I don't think they think like that, but that is how it is. People (students) often come to the levels when they are having more sickness which everybody recognises as being a sign of stress, and even so, they (trained staff) would still not automatically stop and think- it has to get really quite far before they would. If you haven't broken down and cried or said "I can't cope," nobody will stop and see you automatically every day. I don't think people look at each other's faces enough to know how they feel.

JG: Why do you think that is?

Tutor: I don't know...perhaps they are going through their own stresses, because at the moment it seems to be that all the people on the ward are going through feelings of stress too, and people aren't looking at each other enough.

Avoiding eye contact is a recognised defensive response when people either 'cannot or will not get involved with other people or situations they cannot manage'. (Heron 1990, p.49)

The student's surprise that the tutor recognised her distress indicated that the student was not expecting such empathy. Why this might be needs to be explored here. To help identify some of the possible issues surrounding emotional expression I turned to the data on Interpersonal skills groupwork in the S.O.N. (1). As stated in section the previous section, it is in such groupwork that interpersonal and emotional issues get addressed. Some verbatim accounts will bring the subject alive:

Students, by sharing their feeling about their experiences on the wards can support each other on the ward, and if they do this sharing with a tutor, who will also share, then they have permission to use school time to share thoughts and values and attitudes with each other. (Tutor)

However another tutor had misgivings about the context in which emotions got expressed:

A large group may inhibit the very nurses who need to work through their emotions about potential trauma on the ward. They need to share in small groups, in a social situation.

Un-prepared people will not open up in large groups. People have problems with coping with emotions. (Tutor)

This 'Unpreparedness' seems to refer to the interactive and experiential nature of groupwork, where people share personal experiences. Nurses, no different from most people new to experiential group learning (see Chapter 1) find it quite uncomfortable to the point of feeling threatened. The reasons why student nurses might find it difficult will be discussed as this chapter unfolds. The justification for emotional education was accepted by most tutors and can be summarised by one tutor's account:

Nurses need to know their emotional competence before being exposed to serious incidents on the ward, and before they can help others. (Tutor)

One of the patterns I observed at interview was that as soon as participants, both tutors and students, began to acknowledge that emotional education and the development of interpersonal skills were important in nurse education, there would then be a shift to a "Yes, but...." and the reasons or justifications for this not happening would emerge. It was then difficult to steer participants to explore in more depth what form of emotional education could be addressed in the School of Nursing. Here is one of the links with the over-riding category of 'With-holding self as a strategy for self-management'. I tested this "Yes, but.." uncertainty out by posing the question as to whether the School of Nursing was a suitable place for students to express emotional needs and feelings:

> JG: Where do you think this should happen? Would you think that this should be under the remit of the Educational Unit, to check out people's capacity to be emotionally competent before they are actually put in situations of emotional trauma?

> Tutor: I'm not entirely sure that it will ever totally come within the educational remit. I think a lot of working through feelings, particularly in the early stages of training will come into the extra-curricular activities. Where they share emotions and explore feelings with each other, nine times out of ten it is done outside the classroom. Educational staff seem too distant, they may be even threatening to the students. The experience and the knowledge and power that is seen to be held by the educational staff, may actually deter them from working their way right through it. (their feelings).
>   I think group support and group cohesion are very important in the early stages. Later on in their training, then they actually feel more comfortable with their socialisation into the role of the nurse, then I think they are actually able to cope with discussing it (their feelings) with tutors.

I reflected back to the tutor my understanding of what she said:

> JG: It sounds like, for newer learners, the educational environment is not the best place for them to explore their emotional state

The tutor replied:

As it stands at the moment, it isn't necessarily the best place, ..from the point of view of their own experience, they may not feel comfortable with that...they will actually tend to use the circumstances which are familiar to them. They may prefer to share behind the bike shed, so to speak...that is, with their peers.

..and another tutor confirmed this when she said:

The educational environment is not necessarily the best place for junior students to explore their emotional states. The environment may not be (psychologically) `comfortable' enough.

These sentiments are congruent with the tutors reluctance to engage with the educational processes as described in the last section on `Living the contradiction' and address the issue of- `to whom' and `how' of emotional expression. Burnard (1991: 152) found the same concern about psychological `safety' in his study of nurses' perceptions of experiential learning in nurse education. (See Chapter 1) The two tutors above seemed to accept that the students may not have been accustomed to sharing feelings with teachers in formal education. This could account in part for the discomfort they felt at sharing their feelings and seeking support from the tutors. They also said that students may not trust tutors or feel psychologically safe because of the hierarchical relationship.

Building on this concept through theoretical sampling of tutors' beliefs about the appropriateness of emotional expression in experiential groupwork, I inquired of one tutor:

JG: One of the things you highlighted was about learning from experience, about how to manage your own emotions and other people's emotions...

Tutor: You need to be in the situation to trigger those emotions before you can learn how to cope with them...and until you have learned how to cope with your own feelings, you will find it very difficult to cope with somebody else's feelings.

JG: Right, and this is in the context of educating students? Is there a place for educating emotionally in the school environment?

Tutor: I think it is almost impossible to educate a group emotionally, although you need the group to actually bring it up, because there is such a breadth of experience in the group, that you can actually perhaps surface the situation and get people to think about it, but I don't think you can actually teach them. I think you have to raise awareness and then they learn their own ways of coping and dealing with it.

The tutor then went on to give an example of a group of very junior students who had been taken to the mortuary to see a post-mortem, 'and it really opened a can of worms' as none of the students were emotionally ready to see a dead body, let alone one 'hacked up in front of them'... it took a long time to rebuild those students. (Tutor's words in inverted commas). The school (staff) apparently learned from this experience about students not always being ready for all types of experiences. The fact that it took a long time to 'rebuild those students' would mean that the students lost confidence in their own ability to manage their emotions and lost trust in an educational system which would expose them to such a traumatic situation. The question also arises as to how this tutor defined teaching. She does not seem to equate raising awareness of emotional issues with educating nurses emotionally.

The concepts of hierarchical power and expert power add two more dimensions to the category 'Learning about self'. The issues of expert power was touched on in this Chapter. I pursued this at one interview by asking one tutor:

JG: Do you think you can support students?

Tutor: It depends on the circumstances, and I think one has to take each situation as it comes. As a Tutor, the pressure of work, my skills and confidence and my ability to cope with my own feelings, all these will help me to decide if I will help another. There are definitely times when I feel totally unable to support students.

JG: Can you say why?

Tutor: It may be that their basic philosophy of life is totally contradictory to my own. It may be that the calls and pressures within my own time prevent me giving time rather than *get half way in and bale out* and therefore break confidence and contact, and when I say confidence it's not the confidence in professional terms, it's confidence in terms of faith within the person, and if I feel that way then I think my role is to actually pass them on to somebody else who can help and support them and offer them counselling or whatever.

JG: So is it more the case of a difference in philosophy and a time boundary, rather than your capacity to deal with somebody else's emotions?

100

Tutor: On the surface, I would say yes. I think if I were truly honest, if I'm put in the situation the student nurse is in, that I have to work through my feelings and that it's raising stress levels within myself and I have to recognise that if I am stressed then I am not able to help a stressed person

The use of the phrase *get half way in and bale out* gives the impression that this tutor has fears or fantasies of delving into others' feeling too deeply and that this needs time she does not have. Also the concept of baling out is curious and gives the impression that the tutor believes that she controls the emotional state of the student rather than the student controlling her own emotions. Again this is in conflict with the andragogical and humanistic approach (which is declared in the curriculum document) which believes and respects the individual's ability to manage their own emotional states as part of their learning process. Yet, as this tutor says, the ability to manage your own emotions, your own stress, is an important pre-requisite to being effective in helping others. This was supported by another tutor:

I think that the emotional care of nurses is important... Again, it goes back to the caring, helping philosophy. If you are not in control of your own feelings and care, how can you care and help another person. *As a patient, it would not help me if a nurse broke down in front of me, burst into tears....* in the fact that I am dying.. and I think that on that score, yes, it is exceedingly relevant for nurses, because very often patients are vulnerable, and they need somebody "strong" to lean on and to actually pick themselves up and be able to stand up again. If there isn't enough strength around me as a patient, then I feel even more distraught and more unhappy and less able to cope, than if I know that I can temporarily pass something over, allow somebody else to make decisions, and they will gently guide me back into making my own decisions. I think that is very important in nursing. (my emphasis)

The emphasised phrase above is based on an assumption which seems to influence this tutor's judgement about how nurses should control their emotions, which is not the same as managing emotions. She also believes that for nurses to know how to facilitate patients going through major life events, from the joys of child birth to illness and dying, nurses themselves need to learn how to effectively manage their own personal and professional life events. However, as we have seen, tutors do not always see themselves as being capable of offering emotional education. As this discussion advances it will be seen that student nurses also have their reservations about emotional education. As one student said 'The group in school is too big to open up to everybody.'

This 'opening up' means disclosing or sharing your views, feelings and values about events to peers.

The size of the group was seen to be a salient factor in educational groupwork (see Appendix B, Andy's interview). Both tutors and students believed that a large group, together with the diverse social and educational background of students, inhibited group identity. The consequences were that splits and leadership struggles occurred in the group. Jaques (1991) would agree that the group size changes the group climate and the larger the group the more difficult it is for group interaction on a personal level. Such issues of inclusion and exclusionare all part of group dynamics described in Bion's (1961) and Randell & Southgate's (1980) models of group dynamics. Such group behaviour seems to result from paranoia and mistrust rather than what is hoped for, which is trust and bonding for spontaneous, constructive experiential learning. Groupwork issues will be described further in this Chapter.

Student nurses are aware that much of the content in Interpersonal Relations training embraces the social and psychological needs of people to communicate, whether they are patients or not. Interpersonal skills training addresses the need for social contact for the purpose of preserving patients' personal identity and self esteem, and equally, to develop the helping relationship between the helper and helped. Students in this study understood this and wanted to learn such skills, however, how they should learn them and who should teach them seems unclear from their own accounts, and the majority were cautious about whether they wanted to learn about such concepts experientially. This 'reluctance' to engage in experiential learning of interpersonal skills was also observed by Burnard (1991) and Pulsford (1993a) amongst others. One tutor gave the following reason for this:

> Students as a group really don't enjoy 'consciously analysing interaction of peers at a social level'. It's something they find difficult. (Tutor)

In theoretical sampling at two other Colleges of Nursing the problems associated with interpersonal skills experiential teaching (within the paradigm of the 'education of equals' versus the 'education from above') came together in two critical incidents. At one College, some students complained to the College Principal that the exercises upset them and that they did not want to be 'therapised'. The tutors in question were asked 'not to upset the students'. These tutors then felt inhibited in their work in interpersonal skills training despite the fact that the learning contracts with the students allowed for interpersonal skills to be taught experientially. In the other College, registered nurses doing a postgraduate short course were attending a workshop on the process of grieving. The tutor asked them at the beginning of the session what their learning needs were. The students (16 nurses) spent 20 minutes exploring in small groups and then reported back in the large group that what they wanted to look at was how they managed their own stress while helping grieving relatives plus their own grief, at the death of patients, particularly children. The tutor accepted their requests, and then promptly put them to one side, staying with the teaching plan previously devised. When I asked her later what was going on for her then, she replied that her priority was staying with her teaching plan, and anyway, she felt obliged to make sure the students covered the curriculum content on this subject from a theoretical perspective, with a patient centred focus. These two examples show that the commitment to facilitating emotional development in nurses seems to be sabotaged either inside the classroom or outside it, whether by unskilled tutors or reluctant students. It also shows a consequence for students of trying to combine 'The Two Educations'.

The category of 'Learning about self' and the core category of 'With-holding self as a strategy for self-management' can be seen in a number of ways in this section of emotional education. Some of the main characteristics are:

◊ Emotional expression and competence are accepted at a cognitive level as part of nurse education by tutors but the means by which these are learned are left to chance.

◊ The link between emotional expression and experiential learning of interpersonal skills in groupwork is accepted by tutors and students; however how or who should facilitate this learning is not clear.

◊ The link between groupwork and the structure and dynamics of the learning set is in place but needs to be developed more. The 'where is it best to share feelings?' and 'who best to share feelings with?' is an issue not resolved for this research group.

◊ The link between emotional education, learning about self and the conflict between the 'Two Educations' is made but the confusion and tension is unresolved.

The assumption or the experience seemed to be that students feared being more vulnerable learning experientially than learning by other methods. This fear seemed to be linked with the notion that learning experientially was likely to result in uncontrolled emotional expression to the embarrassment of the individual. This same 'fear' was expressed by participants in Burnard's (1991) research and will be returned to in the next section. To build up the social relations picture this discussion now focuses more on the learning set, looking particularly at groupwork within the learning set.

"Belonging" in the learning set

This section looks at the interpersonal relationship between students and how tutors facilitate group involvement. It is sub-divided into:

- Trusting self and others as an educative process
- Mutual feedback
- Peer support
- Disclosing self to others

The following verbatim accounts are offered to set the scene (parts of which are also shown in Appendix B). Andy, a student, was speaking about intrapersonal and interpersonal problems or conflict within the learning set and how these were managed or not:

> Andy: In psychiatry...if students are having problems you get the whole set in a room and you just say it. You get it all off your chest. I've never seen that on the General side (RGN Programme). You may say, like, well she is having problems, let her see her tutor.. everybody keeps it to themselves. Like a couple of lassies who started (nursing) were really home sick, they asked the tutor if they could have a word, but the tutor did nothing.. like there is no team spirit.

> JG: Why do you think there is a lack of support and openness between the students, particularly when they are in school, when it is just them and their tutors. What do you think happens there?

> Andy: Well I think there is a lack of trust, to tell you the truth

> JG: Lack of trust?

> Andy: Yes, like in our set, it's like being back at school, do you know, so like you have the bossy type of people, the quiet ones and some who just dislike each other. The thing is it is not easy to open up with a teacher, she is outside of the group, even though she is the teacher, she is not of the set therefore you wouldn't open up as much.

And from a tutor's perspective:

> I think we mix it up, rather, now we start them straight in there caring for people, and really they don't care about each other at all, except in little pockets. Maybe one will care for another, but the whole group won't care for one. If one person is a bit odd, they're not even accepted

in the group. If they could keep that person in the group, that would demonstrate caring.

This one section of dialogue summarises many of the issues of the group dynamic within the educational setting; how healthy it is and how conducive it is to the educational endeavour. It also highlights some of the behaviours which influence individual and co-operative learning and there is also more evidence of the effect of the hierarchical relationship on personal disclosure.

The sub-categories, derived from intensive axial coding, (Strauss 1987: 64) (see Figures 4.7 and 4.8. specifically) are properties of the category-'Learning about self' which in turn is a sub-category of 'With-holding self as a strategy for self-management'. These links will be illustrated in the conclusion of this Chapter.

Trusting self and others as an educative process

With reference to safety and trust in the group, some student interviewees identified some of the qualities needed for people to feel psychologically safe. These are: knowing that other participants in the group will not negatively judge you as you display your competence and incompetence; that you will be valued as a person; listened to with respect, and not 'put down'; that others in the group will respect the information you disclose to them, using it for their own learning, but not as a conversation piece indiscriminately. These concur with Maslow's (1972) thinking on educational safety and the qualities he described are relevant here:

> The healthy spontaneous person -will reach out to learn -if not gripped by fear-to the extent that he feels safe enough to dare... The student must be safe and self-accepting enough. In this process the environment (parents, teachers, therapists) are important in various ways, even though the ultimate choice must be made by the individual... (because)... it can gratify his basic needs for safety, belonging, love and respect, so that he can feel un-threatened, autonomous, interested and spontaneous and thus dare to choose the unknown... (Maslow, 1972, p.43)

Safety and trust link together for Maslow and my own experience of facilitating experiential groupwork bears this out. The psychological safety is negotiated and contracted into by the group. This allows people to begin to tentatively trust themselves in the group and trust others. The nature of experiential work in areas of personal and interpersonal development is such that creating a group culture of safety and support, vulnerability, honesty, risk taking, liberty and respect for the person, and personal autonomy are essential ingredients to enable learning to flourish. (Heron 1989a: 107, Jaques 1991: 185). (see Chapter 1)

That the students are self-accepting means that they acknowledge their strengths and weaknesses and they are comfortable with who they are as individuals; their self-esteem (or self valuing) is `healthy'. (McKay & Fanning, 1987, p.1). The self-acceptance needs also to extend towards the acceptance of others. This is illustrated by the following examples:

> Supporting means respecting the other person's point of view. (Student)

The issue of trust seems to have many dimensions to it, both in kind, degree, context, consequence and co-variances. There is the notion that a group needs to be cohesive for enough trust to be generated so that people feel `safe' to learn experientially about personal and interpersonal development. Some tutors believed that cohesion was an essential pre-requisite for interpersonal skills training:

> I think group support and group cohesiveness is very important in the early stages, until they have more nursing experience to share in the group. (Tutor)

> JG: Can you say more?

> Tutor: With more seniority and more confidence in their own feelings and knowledge about a situation, they may be able to participate in group discussions without fear of losing control; and fear of losing face.

This implies that the students need `enough' experience in the practice of nursing before they can fruitfully discuss ward experiences in the College. Does this imply that they will have `mastered their feelings' so as not to lose control or lose face? The delay in doing experiential work in interpersonal skill could be interpreted as collusive between Tutors and students not to get involved in work which is vulnerable for either or both parties. (Jaques, 1991, p. 16) I pursued this with another tutor in a follow-up interview:

> JG: Do you think that trust relies on a group being cohesive. Do you see them being together?

> Tutor: What...Trust and cohesion? Oh,.yes. I don't think you can have a cohesive group without trust. It's like any relationship, once the trust

goes...the relationship is over. No, because of the differences (within the group) you can't have true cohesion, total cohesion. Interpersonal skills is done on a one to one basis. I do this with students when I work with them. If they have an attitude problem, on a one to one basis I can say `Please don't raise your eyebrows when Mrs. so and so..asks for the commode after her fusemide (diuretic) (...not again .. responding to my treatment!)'

I checked this out with another tutor by asking her:

JG: Some students say it's a myth that they all like each other and work well in groupwork, what do you think?

Tutor: I agree there isn't any cohesion in groups or group learning in sets. Which is the one place where we try to teach interpersonal skill, the one place where we need trust to be able to teach it.
The disadvantage with group disclosure is the lack of trust. In nursing there is an incredible lack of trust because there is an incredible grapevine. In the end the whole hospital knows, we have all come across it. Also there is the fear of loosing face, not wanting to let themselves down with any skeletons in the cupboard.

JG: ..losing face..what behaviour would indicate that?

Tutor: Well, the sudden bursting into tears in public, appearing weak or rushing off out of the room (classroom).

JG: What significance does that have?

Tutor: People (nurses) don't like to lose face. People like to put on a good face and to feel in control. A lot of taboos are still needed to be discussed in society at large to enable people to discuss them as they should do in the educational setting within nursing.

When asked to clarify the above statement, the tutor referred to the fact that people in society do not like to talk of dying and death and to show their feelings, especially crying in public, and it is difficult and even unfair to expect it of student nurses, particularly junior students.

This tutor also saw group learning with personal disclosure of feelings and attitudes to be ineffectual and unnecessarily threatening. She referred to the `incredible grapevine' which in her experience existed in nursing and which was very damaging. The grapevine is about the gossip that goes on among nurses in general, and as such is likely no different from other working groups, except that professional ethic demands confidentiality and discretion in disclosing patient information only to those needing to know for the purpose of treatment, care and the law. (UKCC, 1984) Yet, nurses seem unaware that when they talk to each other about patients and their diagnosis, in the canteen or in Halls of Residences they are breaking confidentiality. Because they are talking among themselves they do not perceive confidentiality to be an issue. Nurses seem to accept this form of talk about patients and do not generally challenge it, yet they do not want the same rules of slack confidentiality to apply to them.

Another form of vulnerability is the notion of `self-consciousness', that is, embarrassment with one's own self-presentation to a painful degree. (Sartre 1956). Losing face and the loss of (emotional) control seem to be synonymous. It seems to be about showing your vulnerability, and losing dignity, that is, people who cry are not seen to be coping well, they are seen as vulnerable and weak and 'letting themselves down'. There is no distinction made between the students showing they are upset on the wards and in the School of Nursing. There is no permission to cry in front of others in either place. This concurs with Burnard's (1991) study on experiential learning and the uncertainty about emotional expression by tutors and to a lesser degree by students.

In experiential exercises a student may feel objectified, non-human, and experience being observed with a critical eye by both tutor and peers. So, loss of face is as likely to be due to embarrassment at practising counselling/ social skills in front of your peers, and the thought of `getting it wrong' and being laughed at, as it is about emotional control. Embarrassment was seen to be a concern for students doing experiential sessions in Burnard's (1991, p157) study, to the point that it seemed `to impede people in taking part in experiential groupwork'.

The issue of trust was such a strong salient feature in open coding that it seemed a causal condition governing whether or not people defined their experiences as educative or not. For this reason it is both part of the category of *With-holding self as a strategy for self-management* and has dimensions in its own right which influences the degree of with-holding. Within the educational context the characteristics of trust were linked with;

- people's anxiety about what others might do with the information they gained about them. Would the information spread around the School of Nursing and even around `the whole hospital' or would it be contained within the group in a respectful way?

- the amount and level of personal disclosure which would be determined by how individuals took the risk of trusting others to keep confidentiality

- the group size, ie, the larger the group the more difficult it is to 'know group members enough' to be cohesive, (Jaques, 1991, pp.20-21) that is, be a group which emotionally bonds in mutual support, to allow for risk taking in disclosing personal issues

- the ability to give and receive educative feedback, (that is, the sharing of impressions/ perceptions of how you are as a person and how you function in your role in the learning group).

- the authoritative status of the tutor and how the tutor role-modelled an enabling relationship

- the level of self-awareness of individuals.

Some of the above concepts linked as integrative diagrams showing 'conceptual relationships between different theoretical memos'. (Strauss and Corbin, 1990, pp.220-222) For example:

Figure 4.4 Internal variables linked with trust

Some necessary conditions and co-variants linked with trust as perceived by participants:

Figure 4.3 shows that trust starts with the individual. The stronger the self-esteem the less troubled the person is about 'losing face' as he/she sees all behaviours whether seemingly correct or incorrect as learning opportunities and he/ she is open to experimenting. (see Appendix F in Gregory 1994)

Figure 4.4. extends the concept from an internal variables linked to trust to the external shared interpersonal variables.

Figure 4.5 External variables influencing trust

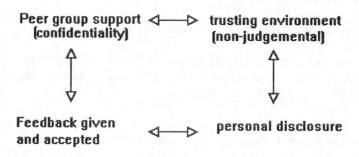

This diagram will be built up after further discussion on the key concepts identified.

Mutual feedback.

This research highlighted that mutual feedback was one of the most difficult issues for nurses in their working relationship. What follows in order to illustrate the point is a selection of verbatim accounts:

> Nurses are afraid that they will be put down by other nurses, so they avoid giving feedback or validation so that it is not given to them in return. (Tutor)

110

> Nurses do not have confidence to give each other feedback. There is fear of rejection. (another Tutor)

The theme carries on in many interviews:

> Nurses are not enabling for each other. They do not support each other on a psychological level even if they support each other as a team on a practical level. It's about self-awareness. Students find it very difficult to say positive things about each other. (Student)
>
> JG: Why do you think that is?
>
> They don't want positive things said about themselves. They don't believe it.

Feedback can mean `knowledge of results' of being or performance, (Annett 1969), which can be informative, non-evaluative, or evaluative, retrospective or immediate. According to Heron (1990, p.41) feedback can `be ascriptive, descriptive, interpretative, educative, (highlighting ignorance and the need to learn) and is a subjective impression the observer has of the other(s)'.

For nurses in this research, feedback of `knowledge of results' seemed to be given and received in the form of criticism:

> Nurses find it easier to criticise each other rather than to praise each other. (Student)
>
> They don't believe each other (the students) when they say positive things about each other.. (in class). Nurses don't believe positive things about themselves. They also devalue positive feedback to others by the manner in which they say it. (Tutor)

These comments seem to indicate a low self esteem in the students. (see Gregory 1994) They appear not to value themselves much because when peers give them positive feedback they are looking for the sting-in-the-tail. The cynicism shouts out at you both from their interviews and from their non-verbal behaviour of shrugging their shoulders in a `such is life' attitude. It is certainly the case that an individual needs to have a strong self image to exercise her or his ability to give and receive feedback. Students do not seem to discriminate between constructive feedback, being criticised by others who are in a supervisory / managerial position, or being criticised from an aggressive stance. From the data, it would seem that both tutors and students see constructive feedback as a form of reprimand or unilateral confrontation which is an attack on them personally. This is possibly a social phenomenon carried

111

over from family and previous school experiences, when praise might have been conditional on performance with valuing of the individual subsumed within the performance. The idea of positive regard for the person, regardless of behaviour, seems still very alien to most people. In professional life it may even be the culture to only give thanks and praise for exceptionally good work with all other feedback given as criticism.

It may be remembered that I welcomed Andy, a student, at the beginning of an interview with this question:

JG: How is it going for you?

Andy: Fine, I think, I've had no complaints...

JG: And because you've had no complaints.. you think?

Andy: I think I'm doing well.

Such a culture would have difficulty matching their paucity of positive feedback with a philosophy of an enabling relationship. From the above comments, one can deduce that feedback is seen as threatening to the students' self-image. There is a fear of negative feedback and rejection. The difficulty with receiving positive feedback gracefully is that students 'do not trust' that their peers are being authentic when they give positive feedback. Also, the nursing culture may not foster such behaviour, that is, the giving and receiving of validation and therefore to give or receive it could be labelled complacent or 'posing'. According to one student, most students see giving feedback as part of the School of Nursing training, part of interactive role-play, which is not 'in the real world' hence they do not give it much importance. The fear of 'getting it wrong' with interpersonal skills training linking with feedback is strong in practice and will be discussed again in Chapter 5. The concept of giving and receiving feedback as an educative method seemed lacking or feared or both, yet the skills of giving and receiving feedback are important in interpersonal relationships. (For a theoretical account self esteem and the place of educational feedback see Appendix F in Gregory 1994).

In the interviews, alongside the relationship between safety and trust, other co-variants identified were group size and the notion of peer group support with group cohesiveness. The next section explores peer group support.

Peer group support

Peer support could be seen as cooperation with peers in joint learning endeavours, with students demonstrating interdependence in creating experiences, reflecting on these and drawing on their individual and group resources to give personal, collective and professional meaning to their experiences. If this peer support happens, then, I agree with Douglas (1983, p.104) when he states that, 'psychologically, there would be a high level of satisfaction for students, related to a sense of security, predictability of responses and to acceptance of self and others', all qualities important for educational groupwork. Peer or work groups are strong reference groups in that they teach and and show approval ofwhat is acceptable behaviour for that group, both implicitly and explicitly. (Douglas, 1983). When such learning is done in a supportive climate it will deepen the bonding and sense of identity of the learning group. Kagan in Kagen et al (1986, p.291) goes so far as to say that this level of co-operation of all those involved in the experiential learning is 'imperative in interpersonal skills training'. The important question being; What evidence is there in this research of links with trust, acceptance of self and others and co-operation with peers in educational endeavour? How is that manifested in the learning groups?

Participants' accounts in the main do indicate a lack of support:

> There is not much support in the school set because there is a lack of trust, people vying for power positions.. (Student)

And again:

> In School, you've got people coming from the bottom all the way to the top, from 'O' levels all the way to college level, and people like me, and people from the middle class families, and people with very little life experience. They have got a couple of 'O' levels and come straight into nursing, and others who come with lots of life experience... and there is a lot of bitchiness around and people get two-faced. The middle class students still want to have control in groups, others follow or break away. (Student)

> Nurses are not giving each other support, maybe because they feel ill equipped to deal with peer problems. It's not part of their role..... it's another human being (peers) but they are not someone you are technically looking after and trying to help in that way... 'Who am I to make comments on what you think or feel.' There is a lack of confidence to be enabling for each other. (Tutor)

There appears to be role fixation here, that is, it is part of their role to be enabling for patients, so the possible assumption is that they had the ability to do that. Yet, they do not feel confident enough to share their enabling skills with peers. This tutor recognised that nurses could be enabling or facilitative to

113

each other as well as patients. Yet she also recognised that nurses will not want to use emotional caring skills with their peers `not in their off duty as well' as she goes on to say.

The opposite case is equally pressing:

> I think it is very important to get support from your peers. The group I am in at the moment are all trained (Registered Psychiatric Nurses). Every one in the group is quite supportive, even if they don't agree with what you are saying, all agree that I have the right to hold that opinion and express it. (Clare, a trained psychiatric nurse doing RGN training)

The statements above show that some learning groups have poor experiences with peer support while others tell the opposite story. The important point, in terms of theoretical sampling, is that both groups identified the central elements necessary for peer support which are those illustrated in Figure 4.6)

The negative statements above highlight one of the main dilemmas that tutors in nurse education face, which is not new to nursing. That is, that students will come into adult (professional) education and bring with them the restrictive experiences they had in previous educational establishments and other authoritative relationships with parents, teachers and others. Old distress with which some people come into groups can take the form of repressed grief, repressed fear and/or repressed anger as articulated by Heron. (1989a, p.34) This `bringing the past into the present' whether positive or negative has been my own experience, both as a group participant and facilitator, and has influenced group dynamics. The transference of repressive experience from the past to the present is considered to be unconscious yet directs the expectations, values and behaviour of the students. The same can be said of the tutor, who, unless s/he actively does personal development work (ie self-awareness about why he/she believes and behaves as he/ she does in terms of the psychosocial roots) will likely also react to difficult situations with students in a negative `distress-laden' way. If the motivational drive and the reasons for the behaviour are brought into conscious awareness, then the person is deemed to be behaving in an informed way and can be more receptive to educative processes in their relationships with students/ tutors. The switch from a didactic teaching style to a more interactive, experiential method within groupwork is more likely to make explicit the socio-psychological aspects of the group dynamic which can be challenging and uncomfortable for both tutors and students. (see Chapter 1) Kagan et al (1986, p.291) were referring to this dynamic when speaking of the `special relationship needed between tutor and student within the experiential teaching/ learning context'. Kagan, suggested that the relationship needed to be based on non-defensiveness, openness and honesty on

114

the part of the tutors. I would contend that this facilitative relationship needs to extend also between students and between tutors as well.

The different students' statements about group support throws into relief another variable which needs to be taken into consideration when looking at peer support; that is the difference between different groups of RGN students. (see Chapter 1) Most of the students interviewed were first time nursing students. However, two of the students were previously trained in psychiatric nursing and brought another dimension to group cohesion. In their accounts, this latter group showed a different way of working together and with tutors in the School of Nursing, that is, they seemed to exercise more control over the educational process and they had a more open, relaxed relationship with their tutor(s) and with each other. This confirms to a degree Heron's (1989a) account in that these students had already experienced (positive) educational groupwork, and as a result were more able to benefit from their present educational experience, particularly the peer support. I asked the student above, (Clare) what helped students create peer support. She replied:

> We get the skills of helping others emotionally by life experience, by role-modelling, watching other people doing the same thing.

> JG: ..and where are you with your peer group? Have you felt any support, or caring from them?

> Clare: Yes. I mean, over the year we actually have got a lot closer. I mean in the first year it was a bit horrendous and I think last time I saw you we had a big bust-up in the psychiatric ward and it had all been brought to ..(a head).. so actually everybody is a lot closer..

> JG: What does support mean to you..as opposed to `caring'?

> Clare: ..support from peers is chatting about it (issues) and giving you confidence, or just understanding really. You can't do anything for anyone else..but you can listen.

And when I asked the same question of a Tutor, her reply was:

> Students by sharing can support each other in the ward, and if they do this sharing with a tutor, who will also share, then they have permission to use school time to share thoughts and values and attitudes with each other. (Tutor)

For both this student and this tutor support seemed to be centred on talking and listening to each other. There is an implicit assumption here that students will share their feelings and thoughts with a tutor as long as she / he shares as well. Yet we have seen that some students in the main do not feel comfortable in sharing with most tutors in a group. Now it could be that they do not like to share in the group regardless of the tutor's presence, or it could be the size of the group, or the bonding or lack of it, or the topic, or a mixture of all these variables. Certainly, the 'power' relationship attributed to 'expert knowledge' in the teacher (Jarvis 1992) can not be understated particularly within the 'Education from Above' perspective. Keeping with the need to probe more at the elements influencing 'peer group support' within the learning set, some answers to the questions about peer support may be found here:

> Nurses are all going through their own stresses so they are unable to look at others, see their stress and help them. I don't think we do care for each other. I don't think it is entirely our fault, because we spend so much time caring for other people that when it comes to caring for your friends you think, Oh no..not off duty as well! (Tutor)

> Tutors who have had good role-modelling are more able to communicate the same level of caring about how to relate to patients and each other.

This could be a case of the 'empty vessel', that is, individuals have a finite amount of energy and if it is being used up 'caring' for patients at work, then there is none left for self or others outside the professional relationship. The need to learn human qualities of caring by having experienced them for oneself, seems to be at the heart of role-modelling. However, who the role model might be, why it needed to be a 'professional' one is unclear, but, as will be discussed in Chapter 6, most nurses expected the role-model to come from ward nursing staff. Yet, if you have not experienced caring as a student nurse, how and where does the qualified nurse learn to care for other nurses?
In a follow up interview, I asked a student:

> JG: Do you have a good peer group?

> Yes, we tend to be quite honest with each other about what we are feeling and what's happening, and that sort of thing, we are quite supportive of each other

The student went on to say;

> One of the things that I know we have learned collectively, or we have learned from each other, is to give each other time to say what we

mean, and think, which is quite difficult for me.. to actually shut up
and let somebody else say something..

This is one of the students who was part of a group of previously trained
psychiatric nurses. There were only ten group members which is small
compared to other groups of about 20 in this study. They met socially, helping
each other in times of stress such as a wedding, house moving and family
bereavement. I put the question:

JG: Do you trust each other?

Student: Mm...(nods, yes)

JG: How?

Student: If I say something about somebody else, usually somebody
that I'm working with out there (in the wards), to somebody in here,
(the learning group) then I know it won't go back.

JG: So you trust each other to keep secrets, or the disclosures that you
have between you, that its just safe in the group, and doesn't go back
to the work place?

Student: Yes..I mean and we have had a few crises as well...

...and the student went on to restate how, like a family, *(her words)* they rallied
round each other in times of life crisis and 'celebration', all done outside of
their nursing work. This illustrates that group size is an important factor in
group support; however it is only one variable, another being the self-
awareness and interpersonal relationship skills these nurses brought to groups
from previous experiential groupwork in psychiatric nursing training.
    This same supportive structure was found with an interviewee from another
small (10) post-qualified group doing their General Nurse Training. Some of
the issues highlighted were:

Student: Within my group, the majority of people can take
constructive criticism and that is very important that someone can pull
you up and say what they need to say, and to be able to listen to what
they say and say, 'Yes...you are right.' I think that shows great
openness and honesty and it is important to have group cohesiveness.

JG: Why is it important to have group cohesiveness?

117

Student: Because it will support you. It is important not to feel out on a limb because this means isolation, being cut off from your peers.

So a sense of "belonging" to the learning set seems to be an important need underpinning how students relate to each other. The fear of alienation can be an incentive to work through differences within the group, while still respecting those differences. However, the fear of alienation can also have the effect of emotionally closing people down:

> People devalue their emotions and consider them to be inappropriate in problem solving or work situations, for fear of alienating a friend... however in the process, they become emotionally malnutritioned and lose a bit of their humanity. (Blumberg & Golembiewski 1976, p.25)

Here again is a link between emotional expression and inclusion /exclusion issues in educational groupwork.

Some features particular to this Post-registration group can be highlighted here:

- These students were not new recruits to nursing, they were already socialised into other branches of the profession, in this sense they could be called 'mature students'.

- These other professional branches were psychiatry and nursing clients with learning difficulties, where the educational structures supported interpersonal skills training and a process based curriculum to a greater extent than Registered General Nursing.

- Also the groups were smaller (usually between 10-12) and they seemed to be able to meet collectively on a social level.

These factors could make it easier for them to be supportive and honest with each other, and to be able to give and receive positive and negative feedback, particularly if the 'maturity' included life experience and chronological age, as Andy stated. Yet studies on friendship groups show that they occur most significantly during adolescence when the need for support, identity and affection seem to be at their highest. (Douglas, 1983, p.105) However, this need to belong may be done at the expense of being honest. The pre-registration group with no previous nursing experience has tended to be between 18 and 21 years old. Of course friendship groups start at the level of affection whereas those in nurse education are made up of randomly selected groups of people put together to train as nurses, in fact not unlike other educational institutions.

In this research, the student Andy made a point of saying that the educational group in nursing was 'like being back at school'. It appears to be that student nurses with little or no previous experience of group co-operative learning have the most difficulty with issues of group trust, cohesiveness and open, honest dialogue. I have found this difficulty within both nursing and other professional groups in continuing education training regardless of age and general professional experience. The link between previous educational experience, particularly in compulsory education and adults' reluctance to experience, proactive educational encounters is supported by the literature. Dewey, (1938, p.19) saw traditional educational institutions to be alien from other social institutions in their organisational patterns, by which he meant, the relations of pupils to each other and to teachers, which he concluded were based on imposed instruction and discipline. Knowles (1978, pp.52-55) and Heron (1993, p.14) have also denounced much traditional education, (by which they mainly meant, pedagogy) as being regressive and dis-empowering or oppressive, as did Freire (1972) in his essays on education of the oppressed in Latin America. While I acknowledge the original contributions the above educational theorists and philosophers have made to progressive and adult education, for this study, the main conclusion I wish to draw here is that people need to have experienced co-operative educational endeavour to understand what peer support, trust and honest feedback mean in practice. None of the qualities just mentioned can be activated independently from each other nor in the absence of the individual sharing with others who he/ she is, so this will be the focus of the last section of the "Belonging in the learning set" category.

Disclosing self to others

Disclosing self to others can take many forms, most of which can only be referred to here. For the purpose of this thesis, disclosure means how people express their feelings, thinking and attitudes to others with the intention to inform the other. 'Disclosing' is showing others who you are and is different from 'feedback', which is putting a mirror up for others to see themselves. Having stated the difference between the two concepts, it is also obvious that 'feedback' and 'disclosing' often go hand in hand (Luft & Ingram 1967)

In a discussion group, ward managers and tutors were asked to address the issues of confronting self as part of personal development in nurse education and the nurses' right to 'opt out' (withdraw) from teaching sessions on loss and bereavement. They all agreed the importance for all students, both pre-registration and post-registration to be able to opt out if they wished to, because:

Not everyone wants to be in floods of tears in front of a class..

119

to which another replied:

> It depends what you are having a class on. (the content)..a lot of trust would be .

and another jumped in:

> Those issues come up ..regardless of self-awareness. They are there and people don't want to be in floods of tears...and I think looking at emotive things and saying 'People will be in floods of tears' is not giving self-awareness a chance. These issues (of loss and bereavement) are going to come up anyway, and those people are going to have to be managed somehow, sensitively ... Getting students to use self-awareness can actually possibly help them work through some issues easier than we probably do at the moment, where there isn't any tools at all.

another senior nurse in that discussion group felt that:

> ..some people are very uncomfortable with self-disclosure, but I think we have to look at why they are uncomfortable with self-disclosure. What has happened to them previously, or what do they anticipate will happen to them, and unfortunately for the health service, we're not a caring profession as far as staff goes, and they are terrified that if they self-disclose, one, it will be consensual, the whole hospital will know about it; and also, will management or teachers or whoever take some sort of action because they have self-disclosed some sort of information. And I think people are very concerned about that.

But what is it that is being disclosed? I asked a tutor from the research School of Nursing what was likely to be disclosed and why:

> Role-play, they need to know how they will react so that they can actually prepare themselves (for the wards).

Prepare them for what? This is one of those statements which formed the story line to this research, that is, what is being talked about, or not talked about, but which seems to influence people's fears of 'What might happen?'

So far in this study most of the 'preparation' in interpersonal skills seemed to be about talking of dying and death. This is certainly an experience which some students will come across in the course of the three year training, yet many students did not experience sudden death on the ward, or take part in a resuscitation. Some students went through their whole training without seeing a patient dying or dead. The point I am making here is that the 'emotive topics' seemed restricted to managing patient crises with little acknowledgement of learners' need to prepare for their own difficulties on the wards; their learner status, how they would relate to senior medical and nursing staff and the emotional work they would do. (Smith, 1992, p.124)

This group's discussion highlighted many of the issues surrounding disclosure but the most significant was the issue of confidentiality, as another tutor said:

> Keeping confidentiality shows respect for people. If somebody says something to me in confidence, I will lose that person's respect if they hear it being tittle-tattled around by others..

which was discussed under the section on Trust; to be sensitive to people's feeling state and to be supportive while they express views and feelings about issues they encounter in their work. What is less obvious are the possible effects of 'over-dramatising' the consequences of emotional awareness training. Believing or predicting that dealing with emotive subjects will have people in 'floods of tears' is one way of paralysing oneself from disclosing. The fear of becoming so acutely embarrassed as to lose face or so distressed as to lose emotional control and 'fall apart' is to make judgements about the individual's ability to manage their own feelings. And the issue of crying? Culturally, it seems that for nurses, crying means 'not coping' as inferred from a tutor's comment when she said, 'how can I put somebody together again if they get emotionally distressed.' There seems to be a fear on the part of the tutorial staff about managing the emotional aspects of interpersonal skills training, particularly using an experiential process. Students also expressed the same fear in Burnard's (1991, p.205) study:

> Experiential learning could get out of control... (perception of tutors) could mean that they like to keep control over the structure of the students learning. Many of the tutors were worried about what might happen if experiential methods led to students becoming emotionally distressed. This issue was frequently discussed in the interviews.

Mutual disclosure allows people to know their differences as well as what they have in common in their thinking, and reactions to experiences. Empathy can only develop by 'putting yourself in the shoes of the other person', an almost impossible task to do if the other remains a closed book. As Jourard states:

> ..a person will permit himself to be known when he believes his audience is a man of goodwill (Jourard 1971, p.5)

Authentic disclosure mitigates against developing the 'professional mask' which Jourard (1971, p.184) saw as self-alienation in nurses. Mutual ignorance is often the basis for mistrust and paranoid phantases about what the other thinks or believes about you, the precursor of biases and prejudice.

As the data are synthesised from all the subsections above; emotional education, belonging in the learning set, mutual support, disclosing self to others, the following conceptual links can be made:

Figure 4.6 Co-variant factors influencing self-disclosure in groups

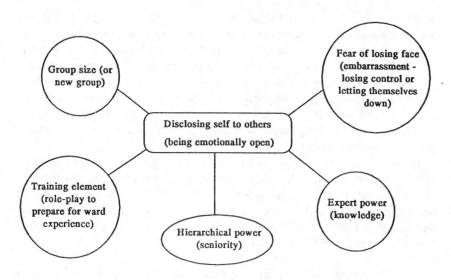

Checking with a tutor what might be behind the concepts of group size, group history (how long it was established and if the students were first time trainees), losing face; fear of losing (emotional) control, which seems to have an inhibiting effect on the students ability / wish to disclose, the tutor responded;

> Students need to feel comfortable, and free to learn..free to make mistakes, and free to learn in their own way... free to be a fool, free to be yourself, free to be honest, to say you don't know, or that you do know, or free to say you disagree.

JG: Free from what?

Free from constraint of the establishment, your peer group,..it is value free, isn't it...from being censured. Free to express your needs, your doubts, without fear of criticism, without being labelled or stigmatised.

JG: Which is the strongest fear...?

Yes, I think losing face, losing control, letting themselves down, is devaluing themselves in front of the group, because they would feel devalued.. it's about each person valuing themselves.

JG: And needing to be valued by others?

Yes, they all feel a need to be valued. There is a need to separate out the student's lack of knowledge or experience from their persona. Their learning needs are only part of them, it is not their whole being. They are more than what they are learning at the moment. To keep the whole integrity of the individual..is important, so that they still keep their own self-esteem.

This tutor had experienced for herself being devalued in a group situation when the teacher undermined her. This experience makes her very sensitive to others in groupwork. I believe that this tutor's evaluation stands on its own without elaboration. My experience in facilitating groups of adults in personal and professional development, including nurses, is that they are more likely to want to be angry, and have a need to be angry than to 'be in floods of tears'. Many of the students I interviewed had much to be angry about, however, the culture they found themselves in gave little if any permission for the expression of anger, so they repressed these feelings. The fear of reprimand was a controlling influence on the emotional expression of students and junior staff nurses I interviewed (see Chapter 5). However, the need to share their sadness and stress was also very evident in what they said at interviews and the manner in which some of them shared their feelings with me. Like Wilde (1992) I delicately danced between inquiry for its own sake, and empathic listening to support some participants' sharing their conflicts and distresses.

In summary, the fear of self-disclosure can now be more clearly defined by linking it with the notion of the self-concept. The fear is probably of personal rejection because the individual's behaviour doesn't 'fit' the individual's ideal notion of how a 'professional person / nurse should behave in a learning group' (the loss of face). Nurses perceive that others will be critical of them for not 'coming up to standard'. This has been illustrated with phrases like:

Nurses should not stand in the middle of the ward, sobbing. If I was a patient I would not like to see a nurse 'break down in front of me, bursting into tears, I am the dying one..' Patients need some one strong to lean on.. (Tutor)

This attitude of 'be strong' seems to be encouraged by the profession, so that it is an implicit norm which gets supported from one generation of nurses to another (Gow 1983. Smith 1992). (For a fuller account of expected social norms in nursing Melia's (1987) research is recommended).

According to some students, nurses have difficulty with:

a)   Disclosing their own fears of seeing serious illnesses and traumas and not knowing how they will manage that, particularly with patients of the same age as themselves. Having said that, the one teaching observation I did where students wanted to speak of their own management of grief, the tutor deflected the students needs to the teaching task which was on the theory of bereavement.

b)   What they want to share, yet fear to, in case it is negatively judged, are their own experiences with family and peers outside of nursing, with accidents, drug abuse, suicide, abortion, and perhaps even separation within their own family, divorce, loss and bereavement.

c)   The training element holds a fear of ridicule, as that entails displaying their behaviour and being open to others scrutiny with feedback about their effectiveness. This accounts for the reluctance of 'role-play' in interpersonal skills training in the educational setting. (see Chapter 5)

The call to delay teaching interpersonal skills experientially until students have more 'professional knowledge and experience' could be seen as a defence strategy, to move away from sharing personal knowledge and experience students already have. Stanford and Roark (1974) found that a psychological distance was maintained by using theoretical understanding rather than personal understanding, and even when the understanding was personal, to use personal cognitive explanation rather than personal experience. So I imagine from the data that the same could be said in the learning group, when tutors talk about the possible problems students might have on the wards, but do not teach them skills to manage interpersonal issues, particularly with senior staff. Such a focus away from 'personal experience to professional knowledge' can create a split between what students perceive as accepted subject matter for discussion, theoretical and clinical knowledge, and personal everyday knowledge. (Jaques, 1991, p.55)

In Figure 4.6 all the concepts discussed under the main heading of "Belonging in the learning set" are illustrated in the following way:

Figure 4. 7 Factors influencing an "enabling" learning environment

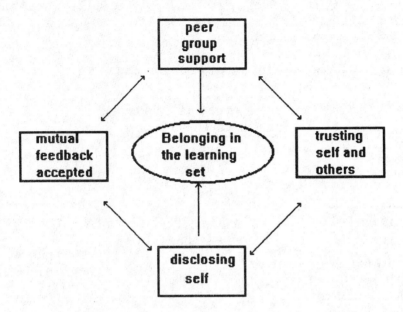

At this stage Figure 4.6 is shown as cyclical, yet deepening with each cycle, as I believe there is a feedback loop going from a superficial level of interaction to deeper levels. One can enter the cycle at any point and move in any direction, thus, a student may start by sharing social information about herself, such as where she lives, her marital status, fashion preferences and so on, and gradually move deeper into more personal issues as trust and confidence builds up. If this information is received with appropriate interest and respect, the student will more likely feel supported, relax more and share how she perceives others responding to her, and so on. Most encounters start at a relatively light social level and will move into more intimate dialogue as trust, support and authentic feedback builds up. The interdependence of the concepts in the diagram reflects a reciprocity which Douglas (1983, p.233) refers to as an ideal group learning environment. However, there is much evidence in this research of disabling group dynamics. Whether this is the reality of the School of Nursing groupwork or the fears of tutors and students which is passed from one group to another is one of the 'What's not being said here' stories of this research.

The categories discussed under the heading of "Belonging in the learning set" have been offered from the positive pole of the dimension of each concept, yet

most of the verbatim accounts demonstrated aspects within the negative end of
the pole. It is this negative end of the dimension that is in relationship to the
main category of **With-holding self as a strategy for self-management.** The
concepts of *keeping a distance, being non-supportive, reduced trust, and not
giving or asking for feedback* are the `interactional strategies' (Strauss and
Corbin, 1990, p.104) by which nurses put into effect their strategy of with-
holding. This can be illustrated with the following diagram:

Figure 4. 8 The negative group learning environment

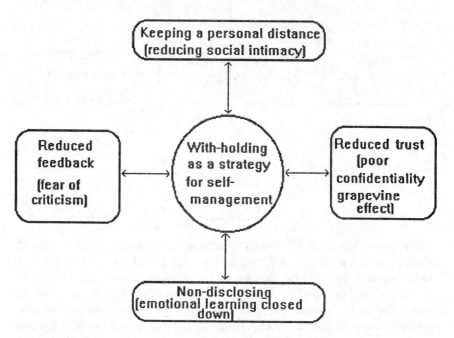

There is evidence in this research that larger pre-registration learning groups
tend towards superficial relationships supporting the "with-holding" cycle with
post-registration smaller learning groups more inclined to create and maintain
the "belonging" cycle. The consequence of this model is that emotional
learning is closed down. This in turn reduces experiential learning which
renders interpersonal skills/ interactive learning difficult to say the least.
Opportunity to develop and share enabling skills with peers becomes
incongruent with the culture of the group which would be seen to be `with-
holding' self. (see Figure 6.10 in Chapter 6) The consequences of the "With-
holding self as a strategy for self-management" in the educational environment
is that nurses do not feel confident or competent to manage emotional
relationships with peers or clients in the workplace, which will be discussed

further in later chapters. For now, it is important to collect together those elements conducive to a positive learning environment which both tutors and students saw as necessary and offer them in the form of a psychological learning contract.

The place of the psychological contract

The hypothesis emerging from this Chapter is that the School of Nursing (1) teaching staff were not aware that they have two different contracts when relating to students while teaching interpersonal skills experientially. These are (1) *The professional educational (formal) contract* to impart enough knowledge, technical skills and socioprofessional norms for nurses to be effective on the ward, which sits within 'Education from above' and (2) *The psychological contract* which is implicit in the relationships that fuel the professional contract. that is, the educational process and within the framework of the education of equals, as described earlier in this Chapter. As Paton et. al., say:

> The psychological contract are all of the attitudes and expectations, some of which may be unconsciously held, which each side has of the other. These often derive from quite deep values underpinning the expectation to be treated as dignified human beings and to have psychological needs recognised; for belonging, acceptance and a sense of identity, which are often not understood as vague phrases until they are breached. Feelings around breaches of this contract are usually very intense. (condensed from Paton, et al 1985, pp.64-65)

For the student this might be to be treated with respect and to be educated in an appropriate manner for the job. That if the educational philosophy is holistic, then their cognitive, emotional and behavioural professional development will be given equal weight, and if not, that they are not exposed to situations they can not manage. All these expectations are part of the fundamental principles of the 'education of equals'. For tutors it might be that students will show loyalty and respect and be responsive to the educational programme offered by the School of Nursing and the wards involved in training. But much of this is part of the formal contract. So how would the psychological contract be recognised? This can be answered to some extent if the core processes identified in this Chapter are facilitated in an enabling way by tutors, that is 'Learning about self', including emotional learning, learning to trust self and others, giving and receiving authentic feedback, and learning to share self with others. Paton, et al (1985) when speaking of the psychological contract, were speaking about industrial organisational contracts between employer and employees. However, the concept transfers well to educational relationships, particularly when personal and professional development go hand in hand as has been the practice in educational workshops run by the Human Potential Resource Group. (Gregory 1993)

The alive awareness and practices of these core processes which are important to group learning would form the psychological contract. The attributes are like Rogers' (1967) own account of an enabling relationship between helper and helped, teacher and student. (see Chapter 1) The maintenance of the psychological contract between tutors and students could be a way of role modelling high quality interpersonal relating with students. Experiences of being facilitated both personally and professionally in an enabling way, by tutors demonstrating honesty and sincerity, who keep tight boundaries about trust and confidentiality and who are emotionally competent and empathic with students, all part of the psychological contract, will create the learning environment conducive to interpersonal skills training. (Kagan et al. 1986, p.11). This can be illustrated with the following hour glass analogy (Figure 4.8 over the page):

The hour glass is analogous to a top down filtration which needs to be initiated by the teacher (top down) and which lays the foundation for a conducive learning environment. It also reflects a positive feedback loop as when the qualities of 'good facilitation' start filtering through via an explicit psychological contract. What is being filtered through will be reflected back to the teacher from the students. For example, for the teacher to have appropriate expert power would not automatically create psychological safety for the student, but is likely to happen if the teacher feels psychologically safe with using her / his expert power. What this means is that teachers need to be competent in all the attributes they want to create in the students through the educative experience. This is the essence of the psychological contract, the students know that the teacher is competent and confident to facilitate their learning. The model above encourages a creative approach to the 'Education of Equals', and would counteract the 'Living the contradiction' phenomenon discussed earlier in this Chapter.

Figure 4. 9 The psychological contract

Facilitating "Learning about self"

Teacher

mutual self-disclosur of feelings, values and beliefs
competent in facilitating experiential learning
role model intentional therapeutic behaviour
valuing/ respecting the individual
good understanding of group dynamics
creative interactive group learning
supporting personal development
appropriate hierarchical power
appropriate expert power

THE PSYCHOLOGICAL CONTRACT

Student/ Group

psychologically 'safe'
feeling free to take risks
more aware of group process
transferability of learning to work
more self directed autonomous learner
emotionally competent with self and others

Learning outcomes

Bringing all of the strands together the concepts link to form two distinct educational possibilities, that is that the educational environment is conducive to learning where people feel they belong in the ways described in Figure 4.6 or the alternative is that the negative aspects of educational groupwork (Figure 4.7) create difficulties with trusting and disclosure leading to sociopsychological process 'With-holding self'. The sub-categories illustrated in Figure 4.1. are subsumed under the category of 'With-holding self as a strategy for self management' illustrated below:

129

Figure 4.10 With-holding self as a strategy for self-management (2)
(shown previously as Figure 4.2)

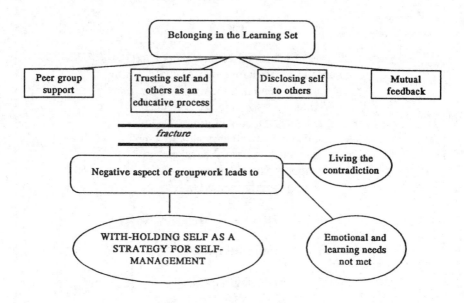

The dimensional aspect of the basic socio-psychological process seemed to be the choice students and tutors made, whether conscious or not to either create and maintain a sense of "belonging" in groups through making the learning environment psychologically safe as shown by figure 4.6 or to avoid that status with the danger of creating the cycle of with-holding as shown in figure 4.7.

Conclusion

The questions which were introduced at the beginning to this Chapter have been explored. It would seem that the interpersonal relationships are rich in individuals' and group expectations, intentions and the private agendas which each brings to the relationship. We have seen that the personal and interpersonal skills training is a delicate area which will be explored further in Chapter 5. However, many of the requirements for experiential learning of interpersonal qualities of an enabling nature were not in place. The question about nurses relationships on the wards will be discussed in Chapter 5.

The core socio-psychological category of **With-holding self as a strategy for self-management** was found to operate for individuals and as a group phenomenon when they perceived that the situation (in the classroom) or interpersonal relationships (particularly with peers) was not conducive to experiential methods of learning about self. To address this sense or experience of personal vulnerability, a psychological learning contract was advocated and developed making use of the participants' own accounts of the attributes they would like to see in the facilitation of learning.

5 Interpersonal skills training

Introduction

Chapter 4 concentrated on the relationship between tutors and students. The relationships were discussed as sociopsychological processes within the educational context, without specifying what the educational content was about. This chapter will dwell much more on the tasks of the group within interpersonal skills training and discussions on interpersonal issues. It will draw upon the theoretical categories discussed in the previous chapter, particularly those of 'Learning about self' and 'Belonging in the learning set' with its sub-categories in an effort to integrate the interpersonal skills content and the interpersonal processes which combine in the curriculum model.

To what degree do the nurse tutor and student nurse need an educational relationship to facilitate personal and interpersonal development and to learn enabling skills for her/his patients? Where do the concepts of disclosing self to others, mutual feedback, trusting self and others, peer group support and the psychological contract fit into the education of nurses? To answer these questions I needed to obtain people's perceptions of the nature of the personal and interpersonal development taught in the School of Nursing as well as the methods used to teach them. That others within nursing see this as an important area of nurse education is evidenced by one of the stated aims in the curriculum document for the three year Registered General Nurse training:

Aim No.5   To acquire highly developed interpersonal skills in order to facilitate caring relationships with clients/patients and significant others and initiate and maintain therapeutic relationships. (S.O.N (2) 1990, p.14)

A definition of 'therapeutic' which, combined with the definition of 'enabling' was offered in Chapter 1 form the boundaries of a 'therapeutic relationship'. This definition has been drawn from participants' comments in this study and links with

Cassee (1975) who found informal emotionally open communications to be therapeutic to both nurses and patients. Looking at the educational processes discussed in the previous chapter, there were many concerns and assumptions concerning the nature of the educational group and its effectiveness as a forum for teaching interpersonal relationship skills of a therapeutic kind. These issues are the focus of this Chapter.

Interpersonal skills training in the School of Nursing

The nature of the interpersonal dynamic between nurses themselves is not usually the focus of attention in curriculum documents, and the situation in interpersonal skills training is no different. The aim of teaching interpersonal skills is to enable nurses to use these skills in their professional carer/ practitioner role, not that they will use them with each other. Having said that, the curriculum document in this research S.O.N.(2) states:

> Aim No.4. Nurses will use appropriate communication skills, develop therapeutic relationships with patients, carers and other members of the health care team, in order to initiate and sustain continuity of care until optimum independence is achieved. (S.O.N.(2) 1990, p.16)

Within the phrase 'other members of the health care team' I would place how nurses relate to each other, that is, tutors, trained staff and students.
Kagan gives a definition of interpersonal skills which is useful to state here:

> Interpersonal skills are those aspects of both communication and social skills that are concerned with direct person-to-person contact. (Kagan, 1985, p.1)

Most of the topics in interpersonal skills training are psychosocial concerns in nursing: the need to communicate effectively and therapeutically and the need to meet the personal and social needs of patients, relatives and other people involved in patient care. The skills to manage these at a personal, interpersonal and managerial level are intended to be taught as part of the nursing curriculum during the three year general training and are advocated as essential nursing skills in nursing journals and textbooks. (Porritt, 1984, Kagan, et. al., 1986, Peplau, 1988, Burnard, 1991, see Chapter 1)

How therapeutic relationships are different from social interpersonal relating is the pivot for educational intervention in social skills training. Most studies consider that for interpersonal relating to be therapeutic (Cassee, 1975, Egan, 1986, Peplau, 1988, Barber, 1993) the quality of empathy is important as well as the intention to facilitate holistic health.   The following sub-sections take the main personal and

134

interpersonal modes of interacting which interviewees spoke of under the umbrella of interpersonal relationships and link these with curriculum aims where appropriate, with teaching approaches and the effect these have on individuals. Therefore the section on 'Interpersonal skills training' in the School of Nursing will focus on 'what was' or 'what could be' covered in interpersonal skills training, The section on 'Group learning of interpersonal skills' will address 'how' interpersonal skills is taught or 'covered' as the case may be. Tutors in this study gave very definite indications that interpersonal skills training was an active part of the curriculum in the S.O.N.(1) and yet, through analysing the data there was doubt that this was the case. These issues will be discussed more fully in the latter part of this chapter.

It would be useful at this point to distinguish between a training group (as in nurse training) and a psychotherapy or a non-professional personal growth group (where the focus is on personal needs and development rather than professional needs and training). Psychotherapy, both individual and group, focuses on states of being; of thinking, feeling and behaviour; both intrapsychically and extrapsychically, that is; how they influence personal and interpersonal relationships. So psychotherapy dwells on the whats, why, wherefores, and therefores in terms of regressed, potentially traumatic issues which have influenced and helped maintain restrictive patterns of behaviour and beliefs. The therapeutic intention is to facilitate personal change at deep structural layers of the personality once awareness of traumas have been uncovered. The training group dwells more on interpersonal, social behaviour. It is concerned with how a person behaves and what impact such behaviour has on the individual and on others. The intention of the training group is the improvement of interpersonal interactions in the workplace. (developed from Miles, 1981, cit. Jaques, 1991, pp185-186). This is not to say that training groups deny the 'what' and 'why' of behaviour, as they impinge forcibly in the work place, particularly under stressful situations, but it is to say that the educational intention is more strongly focused on preparing people for professional life. Therefore the educational contract needs to reflect this intention.

The issue for this research is that teaching interpersonal skills using experiential learning methods, raises awareness, feelings and insights into personality traits and behaviour which are similar to those which can emerge in therapeutic and personal development work. There is sometimes a fine line or fuzzy boundary between personal development with an educational mandate and that with a therapeutic mandate. This makes the psychological contract important in both settings. During the research interviews, the main topic spoken about under the umbrella of interpersonal skills was in fact the personal development theme of self-awareness. This accords with the nursing literature which places self-awareness at the centre of a model of interpersonal skills (Kagan, et. al., 1986, p.4)

135

Self awareness and empathy

Interpersonal skills is about the quality of `how' you do things, how in the sense of the quality of empathy and sensitivity as personal attributes one brings to a relationship. Some interviewees' perceptions of self-awareness and empathy are offered:

> I think self-awareness can be taught, and to be self-aware is half way there really... (in helping to look after others.(Tutor)

and another Tutor:

> Junior nurses need to be prepared by awareness training about potential difficulties in relating to patients who are asking awkward questions about their diagnosis.

> JG: What is self awareness?

> Tutor: It means being aware of what is going on inside me. How I feel about things, what I think about things. Why I respond the way I do in certain circumstances. Even why certain people irritate me. Because if you have actually looked at those different things, you can then actually inter-relate more effectively with the people you find irritating and so on...

> JG: So you are putting together quite strongly communicating with others and a need to know yourself..

> Tutor: Yes. Quality of caring starts with self-awareness. Again, if you are not prepared to look at yourself, you can't care as effectively for others, you won't relate as well to other people.

> JG: Why won't you?

> Tutor: You will see all the other person's errors, but you won't be seeing any of your own (without self-awareness).

I would concur with the above tutor relating self-awareness to social behaviour. Heron (1990, pp.15-16) also links self-awareness with social perception and defines a socially aware person as one who has insight into his or her own psychological processes; and understands the social process around them. This tutor went on to say that understanding personal strengths and weaknesses made the nurse more tolerant of patients' limitations. This tolerance seemed an important requirement for caring as she goes on to say:

> Tutor: Personally I think it is, yes (important for caring). And if you are not aware of yourself, you won't communicate as well as if you have developed more self-awareness. Caring and communication skills are closely related. You need to be aware of what communication skills are, and to be aware of yourself and what is going on with you, in the sense that you need to be able to shut off some of your inner noises.. so that you can actually hear what the other person is saying and look at the things that they want to deal with from their point of view as far as possible.

And another tutor:

> Well. .. the students are doing self-awareness, because if they're aware of their own feelings they can possibly understand and relate to somebody else, how they're feeling, and being aware of themselves,.. helps them to empathise with patients.

..the same tutor later in the interview:

> ..nobody can explain to you what a feeling is, or how they are going to feel....I'm sure that giving them (the students) self awareness, *which they do get,* at least they can be aware of their own feelings (and) they might more easily be able to empathise (with patients).

Thus, from the above, self-awareness may be seen to be about self knowledge, especially knowledge about emotional and attitudinal states so that empathy can develop with patients. This corresponds with the findings that accurate empathy statements facilitate the helping relationship and in order to be empathic you need to understand yourself, and should continually evaluate subjective attitudes and feelings. (Reynolds 1985) In studies done by Kalisch (1971) and La Monica (1976) nurses scored very low on empathy with patients using Carkhuff's (1971) 1 to 5 point scale in empathy skills, even after training. Carkhuff (1971) recommended that in order to communicate sensitively with patients or clients, professionals should achieve high empathy scores. Again referring to Rogers' (1967, p.39) definition of enabling as valuing of the person (or positive regard) empathy and congruence there seems to be agreement about what are the important attributes of an enabling (therapeutic) relationship. When asked what their definition of caring was, most of the interviewees responded in the same vein as this student:

> It's having an empathy with someone. I don't..I mean, it's difficult to have empathy with some people, it really is, well, I suppose, that makes it more

of a challenge really, but just trying to get into their shoes, and then, what is the phrase? get in their skin and walk around in it.

This latter phrase is one often used in explaining what empathy is in nursing, yet Kalish (1973, cit. Kagan, 1985, p.243) explains the difference between empathy and sympathy, by stating that with empathy, the helper remains separate and objective, whereas with sympathy the helper takes on the client's feelings as if they were his /her own. Nurses (like all professional helpers) are encouraged to be empathic and not to indulge in sympathy as they could become too confluent with their patients, that is, not differentiating their own emotions from their patients' and possibly counter-transferentially working with patients' feelings as though they were their own, which is considered to be unhelpful both for the nurse and the patient. This is the reason why helpers are encouraged to understand themselves and work with their own emotions so that they can be less distress-driven when helping others. Kagan, et. al., (1986, p.21) indicate that nurses need to work through their own fears and past experiences around traumatic events which may be re-stimulated by similar experiences in the wards, so that they can more effectively help patients.

If self-awareness as a quality is taken to be the fundamental constituent of personal development, then Reason & Marshell's account is useful. They see personal development as having three interrelated perspectives:

> Firstly, from an existential perspective as the here-and-now struggle with one's being-in-the-world; secondly, from a psychodynamic perspective which views current patterns of experience and behaviour as rooted in unresolved distress from earlier (often childhood) experiences; and thirdly, from a transpersonal perspective which views individual experience as a reflection of archetypal patterns of the collective unconscious. (Reason & Marshell, 1987, p.114)

This study is focused on the first and second perspectives. All the interviewees were certainly very much focused in the present, speaking of day-to-day issues of work and relationships. There was a fair sprinkling of regressive material [6]discussed by some nurses as they tried to make sense of their attitudes and behaviour in the present by drawing on past experiences. Heron's (1992) definition of emotional competence has already been discussed in Chapter 1 and Chapter 4. He also sees emotions as the satisfaction or blocking of needs. (Heron 1977a) He goes on to say that in interpersonal skills training, there is the opportunity `to spot the re-stimulation of old emotional pain and to interrupt its displacement into distorted behaviour .... this prevents institutional and professional forms of displacement, and allows for more flexible, adaptive behaviour.' (Heron 1992: 133). Tutors seemed to have expectations that interpersonal skills training would help students learn about emotional competence and empathy, particularly through self-awareness and from this learning to be enabling for patients. The next section looks at the topics covered to address the interpersonal relationships through the perceptions of both students and tutors. Communication, therapeutic relations and assertiveness overlap as they are all aspects of communication in terms of type and quality with the separate sub-sections showing some of the differences. All of this chapter, however, discusses communication in one way or another, either as content or process or both.

Communication skills as emotional contact

This section touches on three main theoretical concepts. These are:
(a) Emotional competence, and practical (clinical) competence, (b) professional presentation of self, (c) management of personal vulnerability. Some of these concepts link very strongly with the nurses' relationship with patients, and were subsumed under a core theoretical category 'The Ethos of Caring' (Chapter 3) which has been put to one side for a future study. The concepts referred to here will be addressed to illustrate the educational perspective of interpersonal relationships. More grounded theory building of the salient categories is a feature of Chapter 6.

The link with empathy and communication has already been illustrated in this chapter. Further aspects of communication are highlighted here, both what it is and how nurses manage this skill. Many interviewees saw communication as:

> ..respecting and treating people as individuals. It's the ethos of caring. (Student)

also from a tutor;

> Some people find it difficult to communicate with sick people, especially the dying. They run away from the terminal diagnosis and prognosis. Their non-verbal communication could show they are uncomfortable with being with patients. They then have to cope with their own emotions, plus the emotions of their patients, plus the emotions that the situation has generated. It is very difficult.

This refers to emotional competence discussed earlier in this Chapter and shows that managing emotions in difficult situations is an intrinsic part of enabling communications. By managing I do not mean suppression of emotions, but rather the expression of emotions in a facilitative environment. The sociopsychological processes of 'Belonging in the Learning Set' (Chapter 4) and the processes linked to it are significant attributes of a facilitative environment and need to be in place if nurses are to explore their 'uncomfortableness' about being emotionally expressive and in communicating with the very ill, and the dying as well as managing any hostility within the client group. As Gow (1983:10) says:

Of all the helping professions, the nurse is the one who has to 'live' with her patient for a full 8-hour tour of duty. It can be argued with validity that this places far more strain on her capabilities in interpersonal relationships than any other profession.

Communications skills form the major part of interpersonal skills training in nursing. (Townsend 1983a) It is not the aim of this research to explain communication skills in detail except in so far as it impinges on the interpersonal needs of nurses among themselves, both on the wards and in the School of Nursing. Some of the interpersonal issues which nurses face in their work on the wards will be analysed in Chapter 6.

Much communication is non-verbal and is expressed in the personal and professional presentation of self, therefore nurses' perceptions of their professional presentation is important. The issue seems one of protecting self from showing feelings, and being vulnerable. In a follow-up interview I asked a tutor to clarify for me the link between the nurses' uniform and the professional role:

> JG: Some people see the uniform as avoidance, a hiding behind, it's like a professional mask, what do you think?
>
> Tutor: Yes, I would accept that. I mean I certainly put on my role with my uniform.
>
> JG: Why would you do that?
>
> Tutor: It's a protection for me, I think..
>
> JG: Against?
>
> Tutor: Against anything which might worry or hurt me. The way that I feel able to deal with things is by *distancing me* as an individual from me as a nurse..

and later:

> I think it is very rare that nurses stop to say anything to patients, apart from talking about their condition and treatment. We pay lip service to communication.

The professional message seems to be that to be practically competent you need to hide your vulnerability. Yet, in terms of self-confidence, you cannot separate feeling competent and practical competence, as there is a positive feedback loop. This as an assumption based on the belief that the more a person succeeds in a task the more confident he/she will feel about doing it, and the more confident he/she feels about their skills the more likely they are to succeed. The question here is competent at what? Is it competence in interpersonal relations or competence in pretending to know what patients and others expect them to know and competence in hiding personal vulnerability? From this research, the need to distance themselves from patients and hide their vulnerability was identified. Some participants believed that they could separate feeling emotionally strong from practical competence by suppressing their emotions. According to one tutor:

> Yes, I think we need to be able to manage ourselves, don't we? Although, that's not true, there are some people out there who seem to be able to manage other people's emotions very well but not their own. They will spend all day caring for this person whose relative is dying...and then they will go home themselves and cry all night about it... I've done that myself, you know.

> JG: The crying all night, would you see that as not managing?

> Tutor: I'd see that as a coping mechanism, but it's a negative way of managing, isn't it, a negative coping mechanism.

This tutor expanded on the inappropriateness of 'spending the rest of your life crying all night', and the need for nurses to find more positive ways of managing emotions by creative expression, that is, transmuting painful emotions into positive emotional energy. This tutor continues to receive students in her office who come with the same issue of 'going home and crying' and she advises them to distract themselves with practical domestic tasks. However, she identified many of the issues which create the suppression of feelings and the reluctance of nurses to express their emotions with staff or peers on the ward. These issues were:

- self-validation about their clinical knowledge and their place in the team, again, an issue about losing face before your colleagues and patients.
- the hierarchical relationship with the medical staff in particular as well as senior nurses on the ward.

According to this tutor, the ward interpersonal dynamic is caught up with issues of power and control and because of this, nurses perceive that they cannot show their vulnerability. This last point is graphically illustrated in the interview with Kate, which will be discussed in Chapter 6. As in this study, Cassee found that nurses avoided open two-way communication with their patients to:

Protect themselves, as they did not know how to handle it.. (the open communication)... and by such avoidance, their relationship was not therapeutic. (Cassee, 1975, p.227)

From the debate about enabling communication, it would seem that the nurse can appear to be practically competent while being emotionally anxious and lacking confidence about his/ her ability to manage his/ her own distress as well as that of others. Practical competence is about how to do things, not necessarily about how you feel or what your beliefs are about trauma, dying and death. Such beliefs and values can be expressed and developed in a trusting environment. Again the issue is one of caring. To show caring for others is to be emotionally open, honest and authentic in relationships. This is the essence of the therapeutic relationship. I followed this notion of `distancing' and the uniform up with further interviews:

> JG: ..about avoidance,.. and I think you have mentioned it again today, that certainly the role and the uniform is a sort of shield, or facade, used by the person... What are they avoiding?

> I think, you know, it's avoiding giving patient care... and avoiding patients asking them questions that they can't answer; and avoiding students asking for teaching.

So the avoidance or `distancing' is on many fronts, not just in clinical traumatic events, but is also present in not meeting patients' need to know, nor nurses' needs to learn.

Communication is seen as both therapeutic, that is, part of the healing process and also vital to patient care. Communication is also the means of educating patients (which is not covered here) and of getting closer to people, both patients and others. For one tutor communication was seen as more intimate than physical caring, particularly when confronting people whose behaviour you do not like. With Cassee (1975, p.232) I would say it is emotionally very risky, takes a lot of confidence and a need to be honest if one is to have informal open therapeutic communication. In this sense, the concept links directly with Berne's (1964) notion of intimacy as part of time structuring. (Appendix C)

The therapeutic (enabling) relationship

In this research, there was agreement between different people's perceptions of empathy as therapeutic relating. In seeking participants' definitions, I asked one tutor:

JG: What does therapeutic mean to you?

Tutor: Communication can be very therapeutic, can't it? First of all, what does therapeutic mean to me..?

JG: Yes...

Tutor: It means improving a situation, making something better... therapy is treatment, basically, so hopefully it's a sort of treatment, not necessarily physical, that will help someone to overcome something, or improve the situation, or make someone better .. it's treatment towards recovery from whatever..

JG: And in terms of communication, in what sense are nurses therapeutic?

Tutor: I think, obviously, communication is two way, and I think that the most important thing is the listening aspect, and allowing people to express what they feel. When I allowed the student to express how she felt yesterday, she then, having got it off her chest, felt better, and went back to her patients. And it was only because she could share it, you know, halve the burden, ... so the listening aspect in nursing is very important, I think, and very often poorly achieved, ... the excuse being the time factor.

JG: So you think that you were therapeutic yesterday for that nurse?

Tutor: Yes, definitely. She stopped crying. She didn't have to keep sobbing any more. She was able to control her emotions, and return to the job in hand. And so I think communication is therapeutic. Also therapeutic in the nurses' attitude, if you have got a cheerful group of staff around you, you feel better.

Asking another tutor the same question, what does therapeutic mean to her, she replied:

Something of positive benefit...something that makes me feel good....(my General Practitioner giving me a friendly hug when I needed it). Most people would find that shocking, but for me it was very therapeutic. It actually made me feel warm, loved, cared for and probably did me far more good than any amount of drugs ever would have done....

When asked if she could say what would be therapeutic behaviour among peers her main criterion for a therapeutic relationship was people being able to share with peers what bothered them, rather than bottle it up. She saw this 'sharing' as part of the coping strategy which she referred to as `having a moan in the sluice' with a peer about a difficult patient or other staff. So therapeutic would mean being supportive to each other and feeling comfortable in sharing emotions and problems. (see Chapter 4)

When asked how she would identify behaviour which was *not therapeutic* among colleagues, she replied:

> When, whatever action they take adds to the problem or the stress.

> JG: Do you have any personal experience, or have you observed this?

> Tutor: I have observed, where, for example, a student has gone to, say, a staff nurse, and said, `Can you help me with this?', which is a need to be helped, a need to get the caring, a need to have some of the stress that they're under dissipated, and the staff nurse has snapped back, `Go away, I'm busy' or `get somebody else' or whatever, and that is not a therapeutic interaction.

> JG: In what sense do you find peers showing empathy and respect for each other..as we have said with therapeutic...?

> Tutor: I think it varies from individual to individual, you can learn, to some extent, empathy and the way that you show respect, and it isn't just respect for authority, its respect for that individual.

In the course of the interviews, enabling skills, like communication skills and attitude development, were seen to be learned on the ward rather than in the S.O.N.(1):

> Tutor: Nurses demonstrate this therapeutic relationship by actually caring about the way the patient feels, emotionally caring and physically caring, and they give the time to care. So there is a model out there (in the ward) some (nurses) always have time for people, and others never have time for people.

And another tutor:

> Students have to learn how to relate therapeutically to patients by experience on the ward. They may learn by their mistakes, which is going to be a bit unfortunate for them and for the patients. This experience will give them automatic responses to actual situations.

And a student:

144

Communication is part of the healing process, giving information helps the patient to recover.

Caring is seen as a quality in relationships which embraces social behaviour, that is, listening and giving time, as well as physical nursing care. This point needs to be made, as with most interviewees it was necessary to differentiate between nursing care and caring *(as a quality)* for people. These are two separate forms of caring. Nurses can do either or both. In the S.O.N. (2) curriculum documents (1990, p.16) therapeutic relating is always discussed under interpersonal dynamics and therefore emotional caring rather than physical caring. Is the evaluation of a `good nurse' when he/she does both? From the literature on the therapeutic effects on talking to patients, (Wilson-Barnett, 1978, Ashworth, 1980, Faulkner, 1980, Macleod-Clark, 1982, Porritt, 1984) and the quality with which this is done, or can be done, I am encouraged to think there is reason for interpersonal skills training to be seen as social therapy, different from physical and psychological therapy. I shall come back to this point in the concluding chapter of this book.

Attitude development

An attitude is an internal stance or disposition incorporating emotions and motivated by beliefs which can be expressed in behaviour (adapted from Evans, 1978). Despite the fact that the tutors said they did not teach interpersonal skills experientially, both they and the students spoke of attitude development as important and spoke as though such issues needed to be addressed:

> Students should learn more about attitude development to help create supportive learning on the ward. (Tutor)

> Mentors / Supervisors working with students are the right people to teach (raise awareness) of students attitudinal behaviour on the wards...(rather than the group in school) (Tutor)

> I see a lot of nurses' coping strategies, on duty and off: the degree of avoidance, the unpopular patient, the patient whom they feel uncomfortable with, so patients don't get much attention. Nurses chatter among themselves. (Tutor)

In the above accounts, there is a mixture of what nurses should know about attitudes to facilitate their own learning as well as illustrating attitudes which were considered inappropriate in a nurse.

The observation on two of the three wards when nurses `disappeared off the ward' when the physical nursing care was done indicated an attitude which is difficult to define. I explained my observation to a group of trained nurses at a seminar and asked them what might be their explanation. The whole group of 20 people said that the nurses were entitled to have a break when the `work' was done. This concurred with the explanation given by one of the nurses on the observation ward, who said that the nurses were having a rest break. The question I asked then was, what happens to nursing when the physical tasks of nursing were finished? This was particularly interesting to know as all interviewees when asked, `What does nursing mean to you?' answered that it was the quality of the interpersonal relationship they had with the patient and his family. It would seem that most nurses have their `interpersonal relating' while doing tasks to patients and then move away from the patients, either to `shuffle papers in the office' according to one tutor, or they have a `well earned' break. Many nurses saw this behaviour as avoidance from social or emotional contact with patients. Attitudes among nurses themselves will be more clearly highlighted in Chapter 6 with the discussion of the working relationship.

It would seem from this research that there is a conflict of opinion about who is best able to facilitate attitude change in nurses and where that might best be done. One tutor (Chapter 4) thought that the School of Nursing was the best place to teach attitudes development while others believed that it should occur on the ward through role modelling by nurse practitioners on a one-to-one basis. The role of the mentor is supported in the curriculum document (S.O.N. (2) 1990) and there seemed general agreement from the tutors that the mentors were the best people to `pick up' attitudes at work, and yet, one tutor speculated that trained staff would be either too busy or otherwise reluctant to engage in attitude education. This issue is related to the teaching environment on the wards and will be discussed more fully in the Chapter 6. The last word in this section goes to a tutor who reflected well the dilemma of how attitudes should be taught or changed and by whom:

> Changing attitude by videoing is not what I mean. By the time we get the student back in to try to teach values and attitudes, a lot has been taught already. It's a question of changing, you can change attitudes or help people to change their attitudes, but, it's much more difficult to change attitudes than to teach it in the first place. (Tutor)

Assertiveness training

Most interviewees mentioned assertiveness in one form or another when speaking about interpersonal skills training in the S.O.N.(1) and the interpersonal dynamic between themselves and their senior /junior colleagues on the ward. It would seem important to spend some time on this topic from the educational perspective, as many expressed strong views about assertiveness training as part of nurse education, whilst at the same time keeping in mind that the assertive behaviour which students

146

and tutors highlighted were situation specific and mostly confined to the hospital wards.

Assertiveness, as an interpersonal quality, is firstly a property of the individual's self esteem. (Gregory, 1994, Appendix F) The non-assertive person takes up an existential position (a belief about self) of self depreciation and as a result manifests behaviour which is over-compensatory, that is, either aggressive, manipulative or under-valuing, manifesting as passive or timid behaviour.

This student's account illustrates the problem when trained staff want to engage in poor practice while the student does not:

> A typical example is doing the drug rounds, where the staff nurse was actually leaving the drugs on the bedside table, and not giving them to the patient, and then saying "Why haven't you signed the card?" and I'd say, "Well, I'd rather wait until she has taken them, the drugs, ..I'll go and give them..

> No, no, no, just move on (staff nurse reply).

> Student: And I refused to sign it. And unfortunately, it obviously got.. staff nurse angry , I was tactful at the time, I sort of said, "Well, look, if the tutor comes on (the ward) right now, I've just had my drug assessment, the whole idea of going through a drug assessment was to go through all these procedures, and we are not allowed to do it.

This student felt a need to have recourse to the authoritative presence of her tutor to justify her stance. This enabled her to think she had the right to assert that she would not comply with unsafe practice. There were many incidents of students particularly, but also of junior trained staff, where the `right to make a stand' about good or poor nursing practice was a real dilemma. Whatever decision they made had repercussions they did not like, either for themselves or their patients. Interviewees' perceptions of what assertiveness meant and how it could be used by nurses showed a general bias in favour of assertion skills, but with much uncertainty and misgivings about its place in the nursing curriculum:

> I'm not sure which is the best way to learn such assertion skills, by trial and error or taught in the School - must one be blind before one can see? (Tutor)

And Andy - the student:

> Learning assertiveness is useful, but the teacher must be good, but inner strength is more important, which is self acquired, not taught. It's strange, on the one hand you get...is with the power, in some ways nurses are

assertive, yet, in others, they are very subservient and wanting to serve, or whether they came into nursing because they wanted power, I'll never know. Its a dichotomy.

The inner strength which Andy refers to could be the self-confidence which comes from self-valuing mentioned in Chapter 4. The concept of power and control will be covered in Chapter 6.

Exploring a post-registered student's statement that student nurses' opinions are not valued on the ward, I asked her:

JG: So what qualities might be missing in general nurses, that they allow themselves to be devalued, or not listened to?

Student: I think nurses on the whole lack assertiveness and they just stand there and take it, thereby perpetuating devaluing themselves. They don't seem to be able to confront others. I have confronted Doctors, Staff Nurses and Sisters and they tend to stand back and just gaze, not offended as such, because I don't confront in an offending way, but rather, they think, this is a student here doing this, and they are surprised that I have approached them about certain things. The reason that I am able to do this is that I have been trained. I think that there is something missing in the training for General Nursing *(RGN)* I think there needs to be more focusing on communication skills and assertiveness.

JG: What would you say to the notion that if you train nurses too early in assertion skills, they will just go onto the wards and be aggressive, therefore it is best not to train them until they have nearly finished their training?

Student: It is quite a negative view...

JG: So how is it in your experience?

Student: It is difficult to say, ..you just don't run a few sessions on assertiveness and then expect that one can go out there and just be assertive. I think you can teach it in School and achieve a baseline and then the person builds on it gradually. It is important to continue to have workshops and updates to keep people in touch with how to be assertive so that they can put themselves forward as assertive as opposed to being aggressive.

From this interview, it occurred to me that one of the problems nurses have with assertiveness training could be about expectations of learning outcomes. When the School of Nursing staff or the ward staff teach and demonstrate clinical skills, such as taking somebody's blood pressure, time is allowed for practice, using peers first and learning by trial and error, the expectation being that competence comes with practice; the more practice the better the skills. The same principle must apply with interpersonal skills training and specifically with assertiveness which we are discussing now. All stages of the skills' training model need to be worked through, initially with the trainer and in a positive learning environment, where mistakes are seen as learning and not as failure.

Figure 5.1 A training skills model

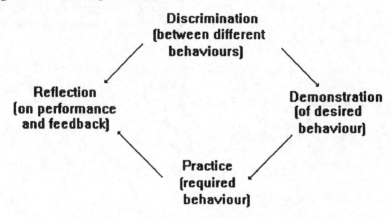

Where the discrimination is between different behaviours, the demonstration is of the desired behaviour, the practice is of the required behaviour and the feedback on the proformance of the desired behaviour is given by the trainer and peers.

This training model is often portrayed as a spiral, as in social skills training there are stages and levels of complexity of skilled behaviour (Argyle, 1969 & 1978) which can be built upon over many training and practice sessions both in simulation and in real life events.

What may be happening in the social world of nursing is that nurses are not given the opportunity to learn assertiveness as they are in learning technical nursing skills. That is, mistakes are not tolerated in interpersonal relating either in the School or on the wards. As one tutor said:

> We taught assertiveness in the introductory programme, to help nurses with stress management, but it was a mistake, it turned into

149

aggressiveness. They (the students) don't have enough ward experience to handle assertiveness well.

and another tutor:

Knowing your rights is not enabling for students in this environment. They don't get a balance. They just complain they are being wronged, not about when patients have been wronged. Some do take an advocate role, but most don't.

Assertive skills are needed, but some nurses have come into nursing to be subservient, and others, because they want power... some nurses push it to the limit (assertiveness) refusing to do tasks, using assertiveness in the wrong way. This can intimidate new trained staff or make them fight back. (the student Andy)

There is a notion of what is `correct' assertive behaviour and what is too assertive which is labelled aggressive. It also seems that nurses can be assertive on behalf of their patients, but not to assert their own needs.

I checked this out with a student by asking:

JG: Did you have assertive skills taught to you here in the School?

Student: Yes, we had a couple of lessons on it.

JG: What's your notion of students learning assertiveness, (and) putting it into practice on the wards?

Student: I think it's a good idea.

JG: Because..?

Student: I think there's a lot of heartache because somebody can't articulate what they want, and I don't think that, given the standard of education that we are receiving, that to be impotent in that particular area is a good thing.

JG: What, given that the standard of education is high, but yet you could be impotent when you go out (into the wards).

Student: Yes, the research, putting it into practice...if you haven't got the gumption (confidence) to go and say "Well actually, this bit of research on....don't actually do anything, so let's get rid of..." If you can't say that, you can't open your mouth, then what is the point of learning it all, so I think the assertiveness bit, and a respect for yourself that seems to come with it, it's vital really, to be able to do your job as best you can, maybe influence the patient's care and that sort of thing.

To check out the notion of `don't teach assertiveness too early' (tutors' comments) I asked another student:

JG: ..about assertiveness.. do you see a place for it in nurse education in the first few weeks?

Student: Oh, definitely.

JG: Because?

Student: You know, we've got a curriculum committee, and I am on it, and I have said that about a month ago, that it should definitely,- they don't teach assertiveness..

JG: What would be your rationale?

Student: Reason for assertiveness?, unfortunately, because of the staff you are dealing with, (on the ward) and I think it helps the student to actually gain from their training, because I think, if you're fed-up on a ward, if you feel suppressed by the staff, if you are unhappy going on duty (working in the ward) you've got two options, you're either going to keep going off it (the ward) or you're going to just grit your teeth and get through that ward (allocation). You are not going to gain anything from it, (leaving the ward) you are certainly not going to gain anything from the staff and it is also going to make you frightened and fearful of going on your next ward.. and I think that staff wouldn't be like that if they were not allowed to be like that... some people need to stand up to them, and not just the staff nurses, but the doctors as well. You find that the psychiatric nurses... they really do stick up for themselves, they don't take anything, they don't take rubbish from the doctors or nurses, and the staff may not like it but they feel quite happy with themselves (the psychiatric nurses) I really think that the assertiveness course is necessary.

This student is making a plea for assertiveness training so that junior students can feel more in control of how they are treated by trained staff on the wards. She also hints that `people will treat you as you allow them to treat you' when she says-`staff nurses would not be like that if they were not allowed to'. Many of the new student nurses also needed assertiveness training, as a way of managing their emotions as `they did not have the words or the skill to express their feelings, so showed their anger by aggression.' And because of this lack of skill, the newer students were more likely to walk off the ward, and complain to their tutors rather than 'stay their ground' and try to solve the problem. She goes on to say;

> It's hard, I mean I must admit after the last ward I don't know whether being assertive is a good idea. But then as far as I am concerned, if you believe you're right and you're doing it for the patient, it's doing them good, then that's ok, but it's hard work.

This last statement implies something else, which is, that being skilled in assertiveness is not the only variable here, the other variable is staff attitude to assertive people. Some trained staff may actively disregard assertive behaviour if they do not like what they hear and see. Such was found by Graham (1981) and Fielding & Llewelyn (1987) who concluded that it may not be in the interest of the nursing profession or those managing it at hospital level to have an assertive work force.

It seems inappropriate that students are having such a hard time trying to get their own learning needs met and also `fighting' on behalf of their patients. One student did express appreciation for help from her tutor when she received a less than favourable report about not prioritising her care of patients with demands from trained staff on the ward:

> But my actual personal tutor was very good. She problem solved options with me as to how to go forward. And she said, "Quite honestly, you've got a lot there that I could take to the ward and make an issue of, because that isn't on" (how I was treated) and she said, "Because you being a mature student, you know the procedure and what is right, I'll take your word for it". And she said, "Obviously, you are worried about the students going after you", which I was. I said to her, "That's not how we should be treated". And she could have made an issue of it. (and go to the ward to investigate). And I said, "Well, look, I'd rather go on my own, and hopefully, by me seeing them and saying something, attitudes may change. (Student)

In this case although the tutor empathised with the student by being supportive and helping the student problem solve the interpersonal conflict, yet, the tutor recognised the student's experience, and showed she valued that experience by not solving the student's problem for her. However another tutor did intervene quite strongly on behalf of a student on the ward where `Kate' is a junior staff nurse. Eventually two students were removed from the ward. I asked the tutor:

152

JG: So it seemed correct in this case for the student to come and seek you out as advocate, because the situation was so difficult, and so the conflict is going to be dealt with by others.. is this the best way?

Tutor: It depends on the student, we have post registered students, already qualified, much more mature, and they will not stand for this nonsense. Most of them are psychiatric trained, they cope with it (ward interpersonal conflict) very differently. They cope with it by confrontation.

This tutor goes on to say that first-students, like ill patients and relatives are not going to confront senior nurses (senior trained staff and Sisters), so it is appropriate to have an advocate.
This is reinforced by another student:

..if the student is very unhappy, then, yes, she should be taken off. If the student has not got the skills to tackle the conflict, then she should be moved. Students' primary needs are to learn, and if she can't do this, it's ok to move her... Tutors normally tell you, if you have a problem, to go to the Sister or the Staff Nurse concerned and try to talk it out.

And from another tutor:

I learned a formula in assertiveness training many years ago.. and I tell it to the post-enrolled students. It's, if you feel unhappy, and if you said anything to the people you felt unhappy about, go back and say it again, and before you do, look at how you should say it....

JG: So when the students come to you, are they learning this because you are helping them or have they learnt it over the years as enrolled nurses working on the ward for a number of years?

Tutor: No, because when they come into this year's training, they don't come with assertive skills. So I teach them this formula. I help them to go back and be assertive because even though I am not so good at it myself, I can encourage them to see how they can do it, and give them the backing to go back and say it in a more assertive way, and then they come away really thrilled, because they've got their point across and they haven't had a bad repercussion due to it.

This is the same tutor who teaches post-registration and post-enrolled students a shortened course to train as Registered General Nurses. Again this tutor sees her role as looking at the interpersonal skills and the attitudes of learners:

Tutor: ...as the learners themselves will find ways of passing exams, we don't have to do that for them, so if I stick to the things that might not happen.. *(interpersonal skills)* and the quality of the caring that they give, that is my main function as an educator, to develop the potential of the individual, the student.. *(Author's note; See Chapter 4)*

And yet the tutor above who became an advocate for her student finished her second interview by answering my question:

JG: Do you think that teaching nurses how to manage conflict would be a relatively useful thing?

Tutor: I do. I think that we don't spend nearly enough time on it, really, and the thing is, we pay lip service to teaching them assertiveness skills, and we don't really do a very good job. The students don't use it, they are afraid to use it because they are afraid of their reports, they're afraid it will affect their progress, their reputation, the job at the end of training. they're afraid of being labelled "troublemakers". So whatever we teach them, until the whole system and set-up changes.. they don't seem to be able to use what they're taught.

Learning the art of confronting and how to take confrontation are part of giving and receiving constructive feedback referred to in Chapter 4. These are important skills of assertive behaviour as well as important in mutual honest feedback:

Well you must be prepared to be criticised if it is your fault. How do you learn to give criticism if you don't learn to accept it. (Tutor)

I will not challenge disabling behaviour until I am sure that there is a positive outcome, unless patients were put at risk by the student's behaviour. Confronting students behaviour before they are ready, will make them regress to a disabling behaviour. They lose confidence. (another Tutor)

This last tutor links correction to positive outcome. She looks to the intention behind confronting and only asks nurses to do what they are ready and capable of doing rather than confronting for its own sake.

Assertiveness is an important part of the management of interpersonal relationships. In practice, it implies that those in the interaction respect each others' rights and negotiate with acknowledgement of the hierarchical and expert power which might reside in one or other of the people in the interaction. Regardless of such hierarchical power, each individual has the right to be treated as equal, this

154

premise is inherent in the education of equals and the humanistic philosophy espoused by this research hospital and School of Nursing. However, as the last tutor indicated very strongly, the ward culture did not welcome assertive behaviour. This point will be discussed in Chapter 6.

This chapter has so far looked at the main curriculum content addressing interpersonal skills. The last Section gave a picture of which interpersonal skills were most relevant to tutors and students, they were self-awareness, therapeutic skills, open 'emotional' communication and other enabling skills, that is, the skills of empathy towards clients/patients. Assertiveness was directed more to the interpersonal dynamic between different grades of staff on the ward and how the S.O.N.(1) viewed assertiveness as well as how they thought they managed the teaching. The final section of this chapter will focus on the group learning of interpersonal skills and links to the issues of educational groupwork discussed in Chapter 4.

Group learning of interpersonal skills

In general the content of interpersonal skills training included communication skills and social skills which were seen as enabling or therapeutic by the respectful and caring quality with which people behaved. This accords with the curriculum aspirations, which spoke of the therapeutic relationship as a sustained emotionally caring relationship. Tutors are in a good position to set the scene for therapeutic or enabling relationships as part of the psychological contract:

> Although experiential learning through the use of diad and triad role-play is valuable, the most effective way in which a teacher can teach understanding, respect, warmth, and genuineness is to demonstrate these qualities herself. (Kagan, 1985, p.204)

In Chapter 4 it was shown that tutors may have a good one-to-one relationship with students, but for the pre-registration students tutors in the classroom were not considered good role models of strong facilitator leadership. Tutors were seen as distancing from the students, not wanting to give time to know students problems (see Andy's interview in Appendix B) and in their own words, torn between covering the curriculum content and paying attention to the psychosocial processes in learning groups.

As stated in Chapter 1 group based [7]experiential learning methods have been strongly recommended in the human relations aspects of nurse education by the English National Board (ENB, the Statutory Nurse Education Body). This research S.O.N.(1) and (2) advocated this approach, for example:

Teaching/Learning Strategies: These will include seminars, discussions, debates, role play, experiential learning and group work as well as directed study, project work and some formal teaching... and a learning journal/diary. (S.O.N. (2) 1990, p.38)

And further on under the Interpersonal Skills strand:

Students will be exposed to group trust exercises and other role play methods to build on their interpersonal skills in order to promote group cohesion and personal growth. (S.O.N. (2) 1990, p.104)

Participatory experiential methods are used to encourage students to explore and understand their thinking, feelings and attitudes, their problem solving abilities and values and how these may enable or impede their relationship with patients. In that learning process, they may also uncover some aspects of their behaviour and attitudes which they may be uncomfortable about and want to hide from themselves and others (Kagan, 1985, p.205). We have seen this `uncomfortableness' with communicating with the very ill and dying. Disclosing personal feelings, behaviours and attitudes can make the student (and tutor) feel vulnerable, hence the importance of creating a safe, non-judgemental learning environment as discussed in the last chapter. In what way does experiential learning teach people to be therapeutic? Nurses, like others training in therapeutic skills can be therapeutic by learning and practising self-awareness, empathy, counselling skills, communication skills and assertiveness and so on.

Given that the interpersonal skills training is taught in groups in the School of Nursing, using, as stated earlier, experiential learning methods or interactive group work and given that much of the discussion so far in terms of processes refer to important psychological issues around groupwork, it seemed appropriate to try to be even more specific about what actually happens in groups:

RMN's *(Registered Mental Nurses)* have learned their interpersonal skills/counselling prior to doing their RGN, *(Registered General Nursing)* which helps them to care for each other more effectively. In RGN we don't carry the communication skills far enough. (Student)

And a tutor:

Most teachers don't like the word communication. They see communication skills as just listening and talking and think, `we didn't have anyone teaching us that and we learned it,' so they don't like to teach it.

However, the same problem of trying to get interviewees to be specific still arose:

> Not all tutors view interpersonal skills development with the same importance, some students will then miss out. (Tutor)

This statement was reinforced in a follow-up interview with another tutor, who seemed pleased to state that:

> Students know what to expect from me. I give them the curriculum content that they want and so they ask me back.

This tutor expressed deep concern for the ethics of creating experiences in groupwork or encouraging students to discuss difficult emotional events which might raise painful or embarrassing issues for them, and is equally concerned for the tutors' competence in facilitating such groupwork. Her fear was of the student losing face and for the issue of confidentiality as discussed in Chapter 4. In a response to questions about interpersonal skills training, one student said:

> Interpersonal skills training in the school..? My learning is self-directed, there is very little groupwork on interpersonal issues. We did one session on 'what would you do if you found yourself on the ward on your own'... That has happened to me when the other nurses left the ward for a meal break. I've been very frightened.....If it happens again, I will tell the senior nurse in charge of the hospital and then leave the ward myself.

and yet another student:

> We had one session on death and dying. A discussion with the chaplain and a Tutor. There were 60 students in the group. The talk was good, but it was very difficult as I had recently suffered personal loss, others were also in the same boat, and found it difficult..

I asked this student if she had been able to talk to any of the S.O.N.(1) tutors about her experience, but she had not even thought of doing so.

So there seems to be a lack of uniformity between tutors about what interpersonal skills to teach and about the appropriateness of groupwork in interpersonal skills training. Students told a variety of tales, most of which were experiences they did not find useful. Tutors seemed to understand what groupwork was intended for, as one tutor claimed:

> Teacher acts as a catalyst in the large group by planting the seeds of ideas about issues of dying and death. They (the students) then share their

157

feelings with one or two people they feel comfortable with. Students will share different topics with different people.

When asked the purpose of interpersonal skills this same tutor responded that 'interpersonal skills should be about caring.. and spending time with each other as time and caring go together.' However, we can see that what tutors say could and should happen does not happen in reality. Why this might be so can be found in the following statements:

> Tutor: What I imagine goes on in group teaching in interpersonal skills is probably my own ignorance, as I have never done any of it myself, so I can't truly say what is going on. Perhaps if I had to do a communication session, research it, revise my psychology, and evaluate these sessions, if the students found them useful, perhaps then I would change my opinion about how useful they are, as it stands at the moment, I am not that keen.

> JG: Would you see any advantages in, if you did have to do a session for students that instead of researching it and looking up your psychology, that you actually went and did it for yourself as a participant?

> Tutor: Yes, I think it would be quite interesting to do it that way. I've had little experience of group learning, but we did something here once, with games to get to know each other's names. Now if there were other games like that which could actually help you to build up your communication skills which you could then use on the ward, well I'd be all for that.

Another Tutor:

> I think using learning groups in School would help nurses gain the skills of caring for each other. One thing that is lacking in nursing is caring for each other.

This tutor appeared to have no knowledge of the volume of communication and interpersonal skills training and experiential teaching material to be found. (Pfeiffer & Jones, 1974, Brandes, 1982, Burnard, 1985, Bond, 1986, to name a few). It was difficult to find evidence of positive experiences of experiential learning in this School of Nursing. As a result I asked some trained staff nurses about interpersonal skills training in general;

> Ward Sister: The School of Nursing can prepare people a bit for ward experience. When I was doing my RGN. training we had some fun sessions on communication skills (drawing exercise) which I found very useful. It is surprising how much we don't hear what is actually said. Most

158

people in the School, know of poor communicators and they can use this experience to illustrate what 'good' communication skills are all about. Some role play might help, but it has to be done properly. Its embarrassing to do role-play among friends, yet if you do it too early, when you don't yet know people in your group, that's just as bad. I'm thinking of a previous training, when two people had to role-play `breaking bad news' about cancer in front of 38 other students. They were so embarrassed. One of them didn't want to do it, and I just kept hoping that I would not be asked in her place. It is intimidating to do that sort of role-play in large groups. It is better done on a one-to-one basis.

It seems that the teaching strategy of role-play (see Chapter 1) to teach social / counselling skills does have its drawbacks. Many informants in this study did not like the idea of role-playing in front of their peers. The fear of `getting it wrong and being laughed at' was a constant feature. And again there is the dilemma of `exposing the students to experiential learning too soon or too late'. I asked one tutor:

JG: Given the state of the art as we find it..(we had been talking about poor standards of nursing care) what sort of educational input can be done to enable patients to be cared for as you want?

Tutor: I don't know..I mean in recent years we have tried to introduce interpersonal skills training into the curriculum, but maybe not enough. If you introduce too much, you sometimes wind up with a very rebellious group. We have seen that happen. The students sometimes get a bit edgy and they get bored with it, (the interpersonal skills sessions). Perhaps there is something wrong with our teaching. I think people get very frightened, they have heard horror stories about courses.

JG: So what is the fear that you have?

Tutor: You hear all these strange stories about people groping.. and exposing themselves, you've heard me say this before.. but I'll say it again,..and exposing themselves, their feelings..disclosure is what I am trying to say. People are very frightened to disclose. I think nurses particularly..but then perhaps I am wrong in saying that ... (I don't know about other groups). I don't know if it is because we give so much, we are always giving..perhaps there comes a time when we think,.I'm not going to give any more... and I don't particularly want to share it with the group. I think that sort of thing frightens people off. People have said that to me, and they have said it to me because I have said it to others. I am not

159

heavily into groups, although on a one-to-one basis I don't mind disclosing. I am not heavily into public disclosure.

This tutor then went on to speak of the lack of trust in the learning groups due to the lack of confidentiality which was touched on earlier. (Chapter 4) She also seemed to bring to her present day judgements and reluctance of experiential groupwork imagined notions of encounter groups or intensive personal growth groups (Yalom, 1985, p.4) of which she had no personal experience. The fact that she shared her anxiety with other tutors, with strong emotive phrases like `people exposing themselves' and `being frightened' could have created a tension around `doing it right'. Such anxiety tends to have a paralysing effect and could create a norm about what it is not alright to do in educational groupwork.

Two other tutors also spoke of their concern with experiential groupwork and students' ability to benefit from such an educational approach, particularly in the early stages of training:

> The new student group have many shy ones and I'm not happy about being in a group doing all those games they like to do now to build up group dynamics. Yes, fair enough, in a few weeks' time it might be ok and it may actually help them even if they don't realise it at the time. But I think it is a bit much to force people into doing these things when they first come to a new place, a new job. I can't see how else they can do it, besides teaching them the skills, because they need to practise them on each other, at a peer level, before being let loose on the patients. (Tutor)

And again:

> Newest students have not really practised communication / interpersonal skills yet. They have worked hard on it in the school with the new curriculum. They have not had enough ward experience yet. They are still finding themselves and wondering what it is they are doing here and why they are here. Some are fairly shy, inhibited people, they have not actually overcome their own shyness yet. However up until now I don't think the interpersonal skills training has made a huge amount of difference. The theory is good, but whether it actually will work in practice, I don't know.

There are many issues embedded in the above comments, for example:

- The age of the students; Many tutors think that young nurses are still too vulnerable about their self identity to start working on their personal development let alone do such work with a group of equally new peers.

- Students are too pre-occupied with socialising into nursing by wanting to learn medical knowledge and clinical nursing skills in order to wear the perceived 'cloak of nursing' with professional knowledge, rather than communication and interpersonal skills which could be seen as 'common personal knowledge'.

- Their level of clinical experience; Nurses' reluctance to engage in psychosocial education may be more to do with their fear of going on the wards with little clinical knowledge, so wanting to learn as much as possible beforehand. A study by Bradby & Shoothill (1993) showed that at one College of Nursing, the first cohorts of students on the Project 2000 course, moving from the first 18 months foundation programme into adult general nursing were relieved at last to be doing 'real work' and be 'real' nurses now that they were more part of the clinical work force. This seems to emphasise that junior nurses still see clinical 'technical' competence as the 'real' work of nurses.

- The other issue here seems to be about the teaching methods and whether students should be exposed to experiential learning, and if so, which ones? It sounds like the issue 'should students be exposed to ward traumatic experience, and if so, when? This reminded me of the arguments I heard when I was teaching interpersonal skills to nurses (Chapter 1) Then it was, "You should teach the trained staff" from the students, and later "It would be better to teach this to students" from the trained staff. Is it the case of "whatever you do, it won't be right?" This fixing of psychosocial education into a double bind fuels the hopeless / helpless frame of mind with which nurses viewed interpersonal skills training in this study. The possibility of this hopeless / helpless frame of mind being a cultural disposition within nursing will be returned to in Chapter 6.

From the above account, it can be seen that there was a hesitancy regarding what kind of experiences the students needed to engage in. However, the occupational needs are such that the tutors have little power to stop the students being exposed to ward-based learning, although they can try to minimise the impact of indiscriminate exposure to difficult situations on the ward during the early training days, before the student becomes part of the ward team. On the other hand, they do have more control over the School of Nursing based learning. How do they manage that control? Is it linked with student needs or the competence of teaching staff? (see Chapter 4)

By the end of the first round of interviews, I began to realise that although I had interviewed many of the tutors in the (old) School of Nursing (1), I had not yet found one who spoke as though he /she used any form of participatory experiential learning methods in their present teaching of interpersonal skills training within the School of Nursing (1). In the main, all the tutors spoke about experiential learning, and the advantages or disadvantages for themselves or their students from a theoretical, or an imaginary frame of reference. Could this account for the hesitancy of tutors to endorse the methods, and why they put so many "if's and but's'" to its application, as the following illustrates?

> A large group (of 20) may inhibit the very nurses who need to work through their emotions about potential trauma on the ward. They need to share in small groups in a social setting. (Tutor)

This is true, especially with a large group of 20; however, there are many ways of creating small group learning, such as 'empathy groups' or home groups of 4-6 people, which could be utilised to help students share their learning. While interviewing tutors and students I discovered that although they said that they did engage in interpersonal skills training, this was not done using experiential teaching and learning strategy, but rather interpersonal relationships were discussed. This discovery forms a large part of the story-line of this research, (Chapter 4) that is, the illusions of what is real and what is imagined or hoped for or feared.

At this stage it is important to acknowledge that the research was touching on three different issues:

1   Interpersonal skills training
2   School of Nursing based facilitated experiential learning
3   Interpersonal relationships among nurses

This three-pronged focus was held, since, although the S.O.N.(1) rarely engaged in self-awareness and interpersonal skills training, that was the only context in which experiential learning methods were used. (Chapter 1) When experiential learning methods did occur the interactive nature of the teaching potentially created its own interpersonal dynamic between tutor and students which I wanted to capture. Interviewees' comments about both the educational content and process in interpersonal skills training are tightly bound together. They are, group size, experience of students and tutors, peer support and so on as described in Chapter 4. The tension between these three large research areas remained throughout this study. What guided the research were the interpersonal processes which occurred through the following three areas:

a   the interpersonal dynamic between learner nurses and tutors in the School of Nursing, as they engaged in educative experiences which raised interpersonal dynamics between tutors and students,
b   how the interpersonal skills training and experiences in the School of Nursing were related to the experiences student met on the ward, and,
c   how students transferred interpersonal relationship training from the School of Nursing to the ward situation.

The interrelationship can be represented roughly by the following diagram:

Figure 5.2   Interrelationship between the interpersonal processes and the educational processes

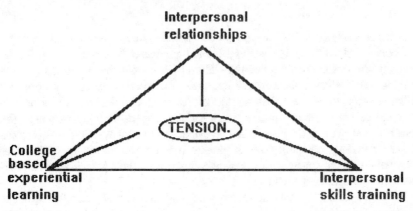

Interpersonal skills training in reality

Going back into the research field, I further tested some of the concepts mentioned in A, B and C above. The findings seemed consistent with what the actual issues were, that is, that interpersonal skills were needed and that tutors needed to be competent and confident in their teaching. There was certainly a tight fit between what the curriculum documents stated and students needs as against what was actually practised in the School of
Nursing. As one student recounted:

> You can't expect to do a bit here and a bit there *(interpersonal skills training)* and expect people to relax and want to join in the training and then go on the ward as experts. It is totally impossible. I would like managing emotions to be incorporated as a large part of the curriculum if this is what the nursing process requires, and the ENB are expecting this of their nurses; that they are able to recognise emotions and be able to deal with them, not only with patients, but with their colleagues.

and:

> It is a very emotive business, nursing, for everybody, but none of us are good at dealing with it, because we don't know how to handle it....talking about dying to the patient. That is what is going to be expected of nurses, so it has got to be part of the training, emotional awareness.

Then again:

> It's not the philosophy of our College to do experiential groupwork. I don't know anything about it at all, and I've never experienced it, nor ever seen anybody else experience it. (a Senior Nurse)

When it became clear that the data did not show any tutor taking responsibility for interpersonal skills training, I went back into the research field with my findings to date, and more specifically asked the question 'Who does the interpersonal skills training here? What is the content? and how is it done?' The answers from four different tutors confirmed that no formal teaching of interpersonal skills was allocated to one or more specific tutors for the number of years in which this research took place and for some time previous to that. Many of the interpersonal issues, including difficulties which nurses face on the ward, were discussed informally with the course tutor either individually or in the whole group when they came into the School of Nursing.

Checking with one tutor about interpersonal skills training, she said that although it was not formalised in the School, some experiential ways of working were taught, for example, the blind walk, which is a trust exercise and some management problem-solving exercises. She went on to say that:

> ..about 1% or so experiential learning was done in the School and about 99% was done in the clinical area which seemed right for the culture at the time. But with Project 2000 training programme there would be less clinical experience in the first 18 months the students would need more simulated experience in the College of Nursing (C.O.N. 1).

The tutors acknowledged that they did not feel confident enough of experiential learning methods to teach interpersonal skills, nor knowledgable enough on the subjects within interpersonal skills. I asked one tutor:

> JG: What sort of model would you use in teaching interpersonal skills?

> Tutor: I don't really know any models..

> JG: I mean, you know, in your head..

> Tutor: I don't think I've ever really done good justice to a session that I've done on communication. I couldn't say that I consciously have done anything like that.

This tutor then went on to say that she only taught introductory level self-awareness and assertiveness, based on her common sense knowledge. Her teaching method

164

was to share her knowledge in discussions, encouraging students to go and practice the skills on the wards. This tutor was very aware of the interpersonal dynamic and of the interpersonal difficulties student nurses faced on the wards. However, like her colleagues she advises students about how to manage interpersonal issues but was not able to teach them interpersonal skills as described using the training cycle in in this Chapter.

As the School of Nursing (2) moved from one curriculum, to a Project 2000 curriculum an Interpersonal Skills Training team was developing. I wanted to see if this team was dealing with the issues which were emerging in this research, both with participatory experiential learning methods and the interpersonal content itself. The curriculum content was the same, and the teaching team was drawn from psychiatry (two tutors) as well as from the Registered General Nurses training team (who were presumed to be already in existence). Only one of the four tutors was experienced in teaching interpersonal skills training using experiential teaching methods. I arranged to observe this tutor doing a communication skills session, after which I interviewed her. This tutor recognised that training tutors in experiential teaching methods was the most problematic, either because their attitude was unreceptive, 'not wanting to engage in emotional work' or the training resources were not available. Also, we were both surprised to hear that the curriculum content stipulated interpersonal skills training only within designated groupwork format during the Foundation program which ended at 18 months. During the second 18 months, nurse education was specialism related, that is medical or surgical, paediatric nursing, and so on when the focus returned very much to the 'medical model' of training.

To return to experiential ways of learning interpersonal relationship skill on the wards:

> It's through the physical manual job of nursing that you can relate interpersonally with patients. Its best to find out about interpersonal skills in the real situation. (Tutor)

and later:

> Student nurses having difficulty in communicating with patients could ask for help, but they wouldn't always know they were not managing unless they were being supervised.

And another tutor:

> because I went through serious illness last year, I can understand a bit more what some of the patients would undergo. Before you were given the theory, but I did not really understand it. To have a therapeutic relationship, nurses need to know what they are aiming for. Trained nurses

165

need to show students that they have this relationship with patients, and some of them have superb relationships.

And yet:

It is difficult to see interactive skills between nurses as they work on their own. Students will find it difficult to see role modelling of communication skills as they seldom work with another person. Yes, Its difficult to know how they could learn interactive skills. However, if a student demonstrates good listening skills when she/he is talking to me, then I can make reasonable assumptions that he/she will practice good listening skills with the patients. Also in passing a student nursing with a patient, it is reasonably easy to see if they are relating well or not. (Tutor)

In fact it was comments such as these which guided me into observation studies in the wards. (Chapter 3) In the event I would concur with the first part of the last statement, which is that nurses do not work together with patients in such as way that the junior nurse can observe the trained nurse interacting therapeutically. My observations showed me that nurses only work together for very short periods of time, when one asks another for help with a heavy, or very ill patient when they needed to be moved. Nurses interact with each other then in technical terms, about the ways of managing procedures and heavy or very ill patients. The observation of Kate, a staff nurse, and the interview which followed were significant in confirming that the model on the wards about how best to relate to others is by hiding their personal feelings. This was done by either showing a `front', that is, hiding a lot of frustration and dissatisfaction behind a cheerful countenance, or by the `busy syndrome' which many referred to when they said `nurses are too busy to talk to patients'. However some of the students found some good role models of therapeutic behaviour on the ward and both types of experiences will be discussed in Chapter 6.

I want to draw together the concepts and issues which have emerged regarding the tutors' and students' perceptions of the issues of interpersonal relating in groupwork and put these along side the psychological contract developed in Chapter 4:

166

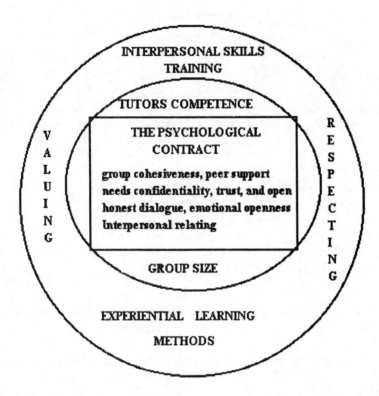

The concept of being valued and respected is a consistent thread. At a study day which I facilitated for another group of Health Care Professionals during the time of this study, almost the same words were being spoken. The group agreed that the demonstration of respect is when they know that people are listening to them, taking account of what they are saying and communicating to them all relevant information which affect them personally and their work practice.

As the concept `respecting' was used by most interviewees their definition was asked for and is presented in Figure 5.4:

Figure 5.4 The parameters of 'Respecting'

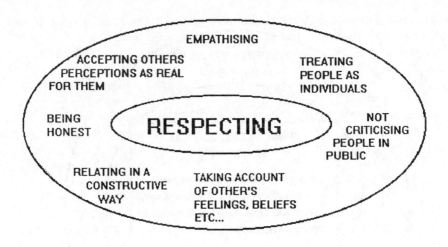

For students, respect for each other was seen as a pre-requisite to exploring learning and for them to feel they could begin to trust. As one student said about respect:

> It is about being cared for, it is about being treated as individuals

and from a tutor:

> If student nurses are treated as individuals they are more likely to be a catalyst in helping others know their individuality and care for patients as individuals. (Tutor)

In follow up interviews, looking at some students' perceptions of their needs on the wards, I asked the question:

> How do you think you are being cared for on the ward?

> Student: How?..*(long pause..)* How am I being cared for? I don't feel there are a lot of wards where you do feel cared for. You feel used most of the time by the senior staff. They use you definitely. A lot of them, *(not all of them)* act as if students can carry on regardless, like robots. I've been on many wards when a lot of the senior staff are like that. Its very rare to get

good support as a student. I don't know what it's like among trained staff, but for students, there is no support.

The need for nurses to be competent in interpersonal skills seems obvious to me from the above statement. Having people working with a mind set which is one of helplessness, as the above statements indicate, is contrary to the aims of the curriculum which is to produce autonomous, self-directing professional nurses.

Returning to the data, it is possible to hypothesise from a stronger basis than when this research started (see Chapter 1) about what the 'resistance' is in group interactive learning in the research S.O.N.(1). Many students thought that the School should be a good place to learn how to manage the difficulties they experience on the wards, yet, for them to manage such difficulties they needed to develop effective self-awareness and interpersonal skills and have the confidence to practise the latter with peers in the S.O.N. as an experiential laboratory so that they can use them with some competence on the wards. One of the most effective ways of making that happen is to teach self-awareness and interpersonal skills experientially and hence the double-barrelled nature of the psychological contract (Chapter 4).

Conclusion

In this study, it has been shown that both tutors and students have chosen to discuss difficulties about nursing and interpersonal issues, but have not put themselves forward in front of peers to undo ineffective patterns of behaviour, nor challenge the beliefs underpinning the behaviour, and learn new behaviours. To do so would mean taking a psychological risk. Such risks challenge the strength or otherwise of the self-image of the individual as we have discussed. So, in interpersonal skills training, the problem seems not so much what educational content is discussed, but rather how such training is pursued within the interpersonal skills strand of the course. The reason why so little interpersonal skills training is done experientially could be explained by the above analysis. These conclusions will be discussed further in Chapter 7.

Notes

6   Regressed material is when nurses experience distress (anger, hurt) by incidents encountered in the ward or School of Nursing which put them in touch (in memory and feelings) with similar distress in the past.

7   The group work here refers to the broader definition given in this
        research which includes case studies presented in groups, action
        learning, problem solving groups and is more in line with Knowles
        (1980) description of `participatory experiential techniques' and not
        just `role play type' experiential learning. (see 1.2)

6 Interpersonal relationships amongst nurses on the ward

Introduction

In this chapter the intention is to draw together the research findings which emerged within the context of nurses' working relationships on the ward. (see Chapter 1) This includes trained staff nurses' and student nurses' accounts of their relationship with each other, and the School of Nursing tutors' accounts of ward working relationships. When discussing student nurses, there will be particular emphasis on their perception of their role on the ward as both worker and learner.

Exploring staff nurses' accounts of interpersonal relationships on the ward seemed important in order to balance the accounts from students and tutors. As staff nurses worked permanently on one ward, it was thought that they would be more familiar with the social and cultural issues affecting relationships between themselves, students and tutors.

The tutors held strong views about their own relationships with trained staff and those of their students with trained staff. Their perceptions of ward relationships are included in this chapter with particular reference to their view of themselves as role models in practising interpersonal skills with ward staff and how they perceived that they could influence the ward culture to be supportive towards students' learning needs.

As part of exploring interpersonal relationships on the wards, nurses constantly referred to their relationship with patients. Students particularly made strong links between their ability to relate in a positive enabling way with patients with how they themselves were related to by other staff. Where these links are important to illustrate the interpersonal relationships between nurses themselves they will be included here, however as indicated in Chapter 1 and Chapter 3, the data collected about the nurse-patient relationship was put to one side for a later study.

The chapter will begin by addressing what emerged as one of the most significant relationships for nurses on the wards: the hierarchical relationship. This was manifested as a basic sociopsychological process of 'Conform to try to belong to the ward team'. The hierarchical relationship was evident by the high profile given to:

- the influence of the ward manager and her deputies on setting the ward culture. This was most evident by how nursing tasks were prioritised.

- the amount of concern student nurses expressed about adapting to ward norms.

- the need expressed by nurses to know who was in charge, and the effect this `who was in charge' had on the interpersonal dynamics of the ward team.

These issues will be covered under the theoretical categories which were developed and densified as part of the process of theory building, beginning with the category of `Conforming to try to belong to the ward team'.

Conforming to try to belong to the ward team

The category `Conforming to try to belong to the ward team' was both a salient category in its own right encompassing many different behaviours and intentions (or unconscious motivation) as well as being an element of other categories which will be discussed as it manifested itself in its various forms, such as: `Fast work is good work', and `Working as a team'. How conformity linked with another core category `The professional shield' through the categories `Presenting a united front' and `Respecting authority' which includes `Hierarchical control'. (see Figure 6.1) will be explored in detail.

I will begin with a sketch of the most salient concepts spoken of by students and staff nurses under this category. These concepts form conceptual elements to one of the core categories central to their interpersonal relations, that is, conforming to try to belong to the ward team. The concepts are presented as a down hierarchy with peripheral (surface) concepts at the top and more central (core) concepts going down the taxonomy. The linking together of the concepts is offered as a hypothesis based on my interpretation of the various depths of the `music behind the words' which constituted the underlying processes linking together what people thought, felt and did in relating to others on the wards. The diagram needs some elaboration to explain the distinction between what was perceived as appropriate hierarchy and inappropriate hierarchy. This distinction will then be discussed later in this chapter. The down hierarchies under numbers 1 and 2 were seen by interviewees to move from what were accepted as positive attributes of `presenting a united front' and `working as a team at the periphery to coercive means of enforcement as one goes down the hierarchy akin to the power/coercive approach to managing change (Chin & Benne, 1976). The down hierarchy under number 3 seems a more normative / re-educative (op, cit.) way of working and when conflict was managed well was seen by nurses to be legitimate hierarchy and gave the sense of belonging to the ward team which some interviewees called team spirit, as opposed to coercive conforming, when conflict was not managed well.

Figure 6.1 Category: Conforming to try to belong to the ward team

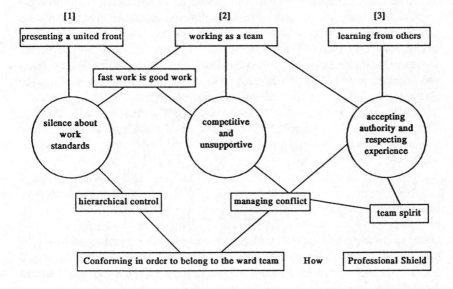

The main concepts linked with conforming will be discussed under the sections below. There will be overlap as the concepts are tightly knitted together and separating them out reduces the dynamic nature of the relationships-in-action. All the concepts in Figure 6.1. have a hierarchical dimension, some concepts forming a basis for others. However, most of the concepts are cyclical and spiral in movement, building from a surface or social level of functioning to a deeper psychological, conscious and unconscious level of functioning. This means that some concepts describe behaviour, and at the same time describe the motivation behind the behaviour, whether that motivation was conscious and declared or inferred or whether they only became explicit during the analysis of data. For example the concept of conforming has many behavioural indicators or ways of being manifested and it is also motivational as 'the need to conform to...' The order in which the unique features of the concepts and their interrelationships will be explored is based on the dominance people gave to the various categories as they emerged in the data. This dominance was nowhere better reflected than in the continual statements about the amount of work and the speed at which nurses felt they had to work on the wards, which will now be discussed.

Fast work is good work

Doing your share of the work, or pulling your weight was a measuring stick used by many senior trained nursing staff to assess junior staff nurses' and student nurses' contribution as members of the ward working team. The junior staff and students seemed to accept this and assessed themselves and each other using the same criterion. According to most students, the ward ethos was seen in terms of efficiency in outcome, that is:

> The supervisor's values is seen in terms of how much work is done, rather than how caring people have been. It's separating.. the feeling part... from... the doing part... in nursing. (Student).

This ethos determined the main priority for student nurses when they went on a new ward, which was, to find out as soon as possible what sort of caring was encouraged and rewarded and what was disapproved of on this ward. What seemed to be valued most by the trained staff were 'performance tasks', which according to Worchel (1992, p.144) require perceptual and motor skills where the outcomes of interest are proficiency and productivity. Implicit in the student's statement above is that fast work is efficient work and the caring trajectory is a 'by the way'; it can happen or it need not happen, but the work gets done. Students need to heed such messages and prioritise their work accordingly if they want to 'fit in' to the ward team. Why the students need to know whether the ward culture emphasises nursing tasks (physical care and procedures) more than psychosocial care is linked with the assumption they hold that psychosocial caring takes more time than physical care *or* takes time away from physical care; time nurses do not perceive that they have for whatever reason. Like Hockey (1976) this research found that time was a constant variable used by nurses to account for the quality of care and attention they gave to patients and to each other, and it was usual to hear that they had little or no time. Beverley makes the link between tasks and time when she says:

> It's a cardinal sin to `stop moving' or stop `doing things' in nursing.., and task orientation is the hidden agenda beneath the cosmetic of `care planning'. (Beverley, 1988, p.997)

An example of what can happen to students if they prioritise incorrectly between task and quality of caring was offered by a staff nurse:

> A student started her day by going round her patients saying `good morning'. She was told by the Ward Sister, "We do not have time for that here". The student was very upset about this.

It seems that the Sister is the one who sets the tone of interpersonal relating between nurses and patients on the ward. This is supported in the literature by the many studies which looked at the leadership role and its influences in the ward (Fretwell, 1978, Pembrey, 1978, Orton, 1979 and 1981, Ogier, 1980, Peterson, 1988, and Smith, 1992) The above student, greeting her patient `out of turn' and who, with this example, represents what many other students experienced, did not meet the Sister's expectations in prioritising her work which was to put the task of physical care to patients first and as a result she was reprimanded.

The above example can also highlight how relationships develop between the ward sister and the student, i.e. a hierarchical relationship, with the tone of the relationship directed by the Sister. According to one student:

> If the Sister is caring *(quality of being)* then you find time for patients, for staff, for students despite the hard work, and the students will say "That ward was brilliant." Whereas in the ward with a poor quality leader, nobody gets time to look after self or others psychologically.

and another student:

> Nurses are still very task orientated. Nurses know Sister wants baths, etc, done by a certain time.

and this from a student three weeks away from finishing her training:

I try to make time when I am doing a surgical dressing or bathing a patient to get to know that patient, but for the rest of the day... you just have a light conversation in passing as you are doing other things. I'm not saying that any nurse will ignore a patient who is desperately wanting to talk, but its five minutes of your time, and nobody is going to come and do your work for you while you talk to a patient. They say *(the teachers)*.. you must give more time to talk to patients, but who is going to do your work? It's so contradictory!

The legitimacy of the hierarchical relationship per se is not being challenged here and in fact it was seen in Figure 6.1. that there is benefit in appropriate hierarchy. Such a hierarchy is not in conflict with the Hospital and School of Nursing philosophy which advocates more equal relationships so that people can more easily `come alongside' (Beverley 1988: 997) patients and each other in their working relationships. Rather appropriate hierarchy creates supportive boundaries for those being cared for as well as the carers. What is being highlighted here is the double bind students and junior staff nurses find themselves in if they have to rely on the ward culture to dictate what form of caring is acceptable.

The above students' accounts confirm that the influence of the Sister is crucial in setting the norms and values of the ward, these in turn inform decisions about whether nurses put their energy and time into physical care, psychological care or both.

These finding are very similar to studies done by Peterson who concluded that although `nurses demonstrated knowledge of psychosocial nursing concepts their care was usually limited to physical nursing care.' (Peterson, 1988, p.85). She made sense of her findings by referring to Peterson's (1983) study which indicated that many nurses are strongly influenced by the norms and values of the immediate work group. Fretwell (1980) also found that ward sisters said they placed the psychological care of patients first, but when she asked them to list the six most important things they expected nurses to learn, specific procedures and techniques were mentioned the most. This led Fretwell to conclude that the "acquisition of physical skills suggested that priority was given to the nurse's `worker' role." (Fretwell, 1980, p.70). If the new student to the ward misinterprets the ward culture the student can get very upset if reprimanded for something which he/ she thought was part of the role of a nurse. The student's need for approval from the ward manager will influence how flexible he /she will be in accommodating to ward norms, and standards of care (Melia, 1987, p.103). This constant adaptation was found by Melia (1987) and Smith (1992), as well as others, to be very stressful for the student nurse. The students' need to conform to the authority of the Sister and senior staff seemed tied up with the need to get good ward reports on personal behaviour and nursing practice while they were working on the wards. This finding emerged from such comments as the following:

Students who are caring in manner, but slow, might have this written on their report, as there is a section on the form which makes them do that. The assessment depends on how the supervisor feels about the person, whether they like the person who is caring as much as they like the person who is efficient but not so caring. (Tutor)

And another tutor:

Some of my students who spent time talking to patients have this labelled on their report as 'slower than most' and slow, which to the trained staff means all the work not done in the morning. So the 'caring' students don't always get the good report.

She goes on to say:

Nurses are torn between talking to a patient and giving physical care...

and:

If I had to choose between patients' physical needs and emotional needs, I would care for the emotional needs. But then again I would never, ever be able to get away from the physical needs, however much I would want to, it's so ingrained in us as part of training.

It was statements such as these, repeated over the past thirty odd years, which raised awareness to the need for the psychosocial care of patients to be given more importance in nursing, (Stockwell 1972, Moores and Moult, 1979, amongst others. Nurse educators responded to such research by introducing interpersonal skills training into the curriculum as discussed in Chapters 1, 4 and 6. However, this research, like that of Peterson (1988) in the USA, indicates that despite research findings supporting the need for nurses to give time to communicate well with their patients, and the intentions of nurse educationalists to teach psychosocial care, the practice, particularly for students in general hospitals, is fraught with difficulties. One tutor seemed to rationalise this by saying:

Patient care is very product driven. People want to get better faster and leave hospital. The attitude of the NHS management is like that too, and maybe the expectation of patients is not to have such a caring attitude from the nurses.

Smith's (1992) research would seem to reject the idea that patients do not expect and want a caring attitude in nurses. Her interviews with patients showed that the quality of caring was very important to them (Smith 1992, pp.143-145), so the above statement could be seen as a rationalisation for task oriented care. This can be likened to Menzies' task-list system which she interpreted as; `an avoidance strategy against the development of a full person-to-person relationship between nurse and patient with its consequent anxiety' (Menzies, 1960, p.12). Beverley (1988) goes as far as to say that task-orientation and the Buberian (1937) concept of the I-thou interpersonal relationship implicit in humanistic values are incompatible. The notion of quality caring is not lost for these nurses, but it is secondary to `getting the work done quickly' so tasks take priority over patient social contact.

The difficulties highlighted here are:

♦ Nurses perceive a need to put physical care before psychological care because of the perceived time constraint,

♦ Because of the time constraint, nurses are rewarded or not for the type and quality of the work they do.

However there is also another possible reason for the focus on tasks over psychological care, that is:

♦ Nurses put the physical care and other tasks before psychosocial care as a way of avoiding more intimate contact with patients.

This was illustrated by an experienced tutor when she said:

Nurses used to be busier with lots of non-nursing duty. Now all these have been taken away and still they seem to have less time to sit with patients, not all nurses, but some of them.

Examples of tutors' perceptions of how such behaviour fits into the ward culture and the time factor are:

..and the Sister has not picked it up that the patient is unhappy, and nurses are tearing around, and the patient didn't feel he could actually stop someone and say, `Look, I'm worried about something..'

The same tutor:

Some staff nurses use non-verbal behaviour to indicate busy-ness, which puts patients off asking for help.

And another tutor:

Nurses seem too busy to talk to patients. They say they are rushed off their feet. Maybe they are rushed off their feet and those (tasks) are not the most important ones to be done. Changes in nursing are that the pace seems faster, but when you examine what nurses actually do, hi-tech, more investigations, none of them hold any sway. It is nurses' attitudes which have changed. Nursing is not seen now as a vocation. It is a job and nurses are more aware of their rights.

The above extracts were taken from the category, 'Ethos of Caring' (Chapter 3) and are shown here to demonstrate how the implicit and explicit norms of 'busy-ness' are enacted on the ward and the possible effect the absence of psychosocial caring (that is, their interpersonal enabling skills) has on patients.

It is significant that nurses did not talk about their skills in communication but rather the need to 'get permission' to talk to patients from trained staff, the 'permission' being the value and reward given to students for their psychosocial care, often manifested in 'doing the little things' of emotional caring as described by Smith. (1992) This is reinforced by a student:

> With staff and supervising tutors, if you get your work done efficiently they (the staff) will not notice that you are not being caring. But if you are caring and equally efficient, they would recognise that.

However, through theoretical sampling many student nurses were emphatic that being busy was a reality, not a strategy to avoid making social contact with patients. One third year student spoke with such a level of stress that it was difficult to know how she managed to keep working on the ward. Speaking about the previous evening shift, which she had found very traumatic she said:

> There are never enough staff on, and the ward was extremely busy. We were taking in everything (patients) from casualty, from fractures to gynaecology, to acute surgical admissions. We were only two of us (nurses) to the whole ward, and I was in the main ward trying to help the other nurse who was even busier than me. One of my patients complained to me that I was rude to her.... because I called out to her to wait... she said I shouted at her. I have never been rude to anybody in my life. I spent half the time in the sluice crying my eyes out, and I did not want to come in this morning, and certainly not nurse that patient again, but I had to..

One could surmise from this discussion that nurses are not rewarded for having a caring attitude if it goes against the unwritten rule of 'fast work is good work', despite extensive writings on the health benefits of social interaction between nurses and patients (Hayward, 1975, Wilson-Barnett, 1978, Evers, 1984, Smith, 1988)

179

Here, the connection between work relations and time for the physical care of patients is offered with a proposition that: the lack of a caring attitude between nurses, particularly student nurses, depends on whether the student nurses are competing with patients for the perceived limited time ward nurses have for clinical nursing work. This resulted in stress, as Smith (1992, p.69) put it:

> ..hierarchical and un-friendly staff relations were still a major source of anxiety and stress for students because of the feelings they generated.

In Firth's study, the lack of staff support by senior nurses was seen to be associated with 'emotional exhaustion, depersonalisation, lack of personal accomplishment and more frequent thoughts of leaving the job.' (Firth, et. al., 1986, p.273). This is a more recent validation of the findings of Menzies (1960), and found also in this study.

In this research, the tension of 'fast work is good work' needs to be seen as part of the tension in the interpersonal relationships among nurses as a group. I agree with Peterson (1988) that nurses work as a group on the ward; however, how they function as a group is seen in terms of the explicit and implicit norms and values which they hold collectively. These norms and values, according to Peterson, are the expectations, behaviour, beliefs, orientation and attitudes of the group members to what is 'accepted nursing practice' for that ward. These norms and values make up the ward culture and is different from nurses working as a team.[8]

How ward group dynamics affected the nurse-nurse relationship is important and will be discussed in more detail later in this chapter. Certainly one way of reducing stress would be to conform as soon as possible to the ward staff's way of working together. From the findings in this research, it seems that there is a norm as to how much time nurses will give to patients and what the quality of that care will be, so that patients can expect the same standards of care by whoever nurses them. Collective conclusiveness seems an important norm, and collective compliance to the ward manager's edicts may be one way to do this. According to Peterson (1988), although primary nursing was put in place for the purpose of giving patients psychosocial as well as physical care, the nurses still looked to the Head Nurse to co-ordinate nursing as well as hold the main influence of instigating and sustaining group norms and values which were then reflected in the type of care given. This matched my own observations over a number of years when I was responsible for introducing the nursing process (Kratz 1980, Binnie 1984) to wards in this general hospital. Then, as now, in my ward observations for this study, senior staff identified patient problems and articulated them as nursing tasks for juniors to perform, with the emphasis still on what the nurse had to do, rather than on the patients' needs.

There is a parallel here regarding the tension between giving physical/technical care and psychosocial caring for patients and 'Living the contradiction in education which was discussed in Chapter 4. The patient centred care espoused in the curriculum is practised at the task/technical level and less at a psychosocial level.

The definition of psychosocial care is best seen at the process level, where 'respect, empathy, emotional openness or genuineness' (Rogers, 1967, Egan, 1982, see Chapter 1) is manifested behaviourally rather than stuck at the level of intention. So the conflict of the 'Two educations' (Jarvis 1986) within the School of Nursing is mirrored in the conflict of the 'Two caring imperatives' within the ward, that is the 'psychical/ technical care and the psychosocial care'. This is not to say that the 'two caring imperatives' cannot operate together, unlike the two educations, rather that in this study, the efforts made by students and some trained staff to combine them created problems, the problems being more acute if the dominant ward culture favoured one form of care to the detriment of the other.

This dominance of a culture of caring and a culture of 'being done to' as 'care' was highlighted in this study when nurses compared care of patients in the elderly care wards and psychiatric wards where psychosocial care was the main 'treatment' for patients, with acute surgical and medical wards where medical (clinical) care was the main treatment. However, there is also evidence, particularly in Fretwell (1980) and Peterson (1988) that it is the ward permanent staff who decide whether the culture is conducive to enabling activities whether for staff or patients rather than the specialism. This was borne out by my ward observations, (Chapter 3)where in the Care of the Elderly ward, because the ward was not deemed to be 'acute' (that is, admitting emergency patients needing urgent medical treatment) it was understaffed. Nurses were allocated to groups of rooms (four patients per room) and spent their shift working alone, giving physical care to eight or more dependent patients. I saw little evidence of psychosocial communication between nurse and patient or between nurse and nurse for the two shifts I was there and the many informal visits I made. The whole atmosphere was so depressing that I found it painful to stay and observe for any length of time. In comparison the atmosphere in the second ward I observed was relaxed, to the point of seeming confusion. This ward was an acute medical ward, with full bed occupancy at the time, but for the most part with patients who were self-caring. The emphasis here was on conversation, between nurses, between nurse and patient, so that the ward staff looked busy with creating noise and cheer rather than 'clinical work' busy. This second ward seemed governed by social interaction, with a ward sister who was young and wanted to be 'one of us' with the junior workers rather than hierarchical and distant. Yet, the case of the disappearing nurses over lunch, when the ward was not 'busy' also occurred here. The junior staff's comments about this ward was that the leadership was weak and the poor management structure did not feel supportive for the students.

The notion of 'fast work is good work' is a value judgement put on nurses' work which mirrors the nurses' need to adapt to the work ethos they encounter on the ward. How nurses (particularly students) adapted to a work ethos they did not help create will be discussed in the next section.

Working as a team

As stated in the introduction to this chapter, 'Conforming to try to belong to the ward team' was both a salient category in its own right as well as being the property of a main core basic sociopsychological process (BSP as discussed in Chapter 2). This section discusses how much of how nurses worked together on the ward was a 'front' for patients as it was a 'way of fitting in' to ward norms. A main co-variant category to 'Conforming to try to belong to the ward team' at a strategic level is the category 'The professional shield' which will be discussed later.

The concepts forming elements of 'Working as a team' presented in Figure 6.1 are 'presenting a united front', the competitive/ non-supportive environment and hierarchical control which will all be addressed in this section.

A hypothesis which emerged from this section of 'working in the ward team' is that: If nurses learn interpersonal skills to facilitate belonging and supporting in groups in the relative safety of the School of Nursing this could prepare them for the more difficult task of negotiating entry and seeking support in the many different ward teams 'they need to belong to' throughout their training. This hypothesis is grounded in nurses' accounts and the synthesis of that data which will now follow.

Earlier in this chapter, a difference was offered between working as a group (as adherence to the ward culture) and teamwork in that the former is understood in terms of collective development and maintenance of group norms and values with rewards and punishments in place as reinforcing strategies while the latter is understood as co-operative interdependence of tasks and skills to achieve common goals through group action. How nurses interpreted team spirit and teamwork shows a blending of the two definitions. Some theoretical coding of verbatim accounts is given to illustrate this:

Figure 6.2 Theoretical coding on `Team work on the wards'

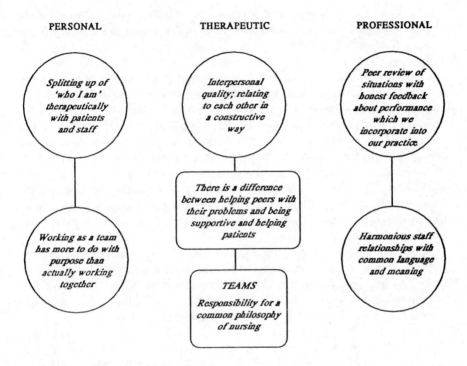

PERSONAL   THERAPEUTIC   PROFESSIONAL

Splitting up of
'who I am'
therapeutically
with patients
and staff

Interpersonal
quality; relating
to each other in
a constructive
way

Peer review of
situations with
honest feedback
about performance
which we
incorporate into
our practice

There is a difference
between helping peers with
their problems and being
supportive and helping
patients

Working as a team
has more to do with
purpose than
actually working
together

Harmonious staff
relationships with
common language
and meaning

TEAMS

Responsibility for a
common philosophy
of nursing

These theoretical codes (Glaser 1978) were supported by the observations done on the ward where the evidence indicated that nurses worked alongside each other, with minimal task interdependence therefore not `working with' each other, and with a preference for working on their own. A junior staff nurse had much to say about teamwork:

> I like to be left alone to do all the care. And if I am giving meals out, I like to be left alone to do that because I know what I am doing. I would rather do it that way.

And later in the interview:

> I like working in a team as long as the rest are pulling their weight. I would rather not be in a team if people are not going to do things the way I would like them done. Here on this ward, you have to ask people to help you. But what is more important is team spirit, like I get on well with the domestic here. We have a laugh and a joke and she will do things I ask her to do, like cleaning the floor, or anything like that for me.

183

JG: So this team spirit, how is it among colleagues?

Staff Nurse: I haven't come across it.... yes, it is true to say... I haven't come across anybody on the ward at the moment that had got the same idea on it (team spirit) as I have.

The seeming contradiction between 'having to ask people to help you' and the notion of team spirit, is not in fact contradictory, rather it shows the quality of relationships among the nurses. According to this staff nurse and others (mainly students), nurses only get help if they ask for it, but to ask for help can be seen as 'not coping', and the request can be resented, so nurses prefer to wait for others to offer help rather than ask for it. The relationship between this staff nurse and the ward cleaner is described as a social and 'equal' relationship with 'laughing and joking' and a willingness to 'do things for her'. This latter quality she describes as team spirit. Interestingly, her preferred way of working with nursing peers is that they should pull their weight, which lends support to some of the elements of 'Fast work is good work'.

The above staff nurse had been working for three months on this ward, her first as a qualified nurse. Her sense of alienation because of the ward culture was still very profound when I interviewed her. The alienation was about feeling like an outsider and unsupported by the senior staff nurse and Sister. The notion of peer / collegial support or the lack of it, was an issue for all nurses. As one tutor put it:

Support is not happening because if someone is good enough working on their own, they are not terrible interested in other peoples' problems. Nurses are not giving each other support, maybe because they feel ill equipped to deal with peer problems. It's not part of their role. It's another human being (referring to peers) but they are not someone you are technically looking after and trying to help in that way.. "Who am I to make comments on what you think and feel" There is a lack of confidence to be enabling (therapeutically) for each other.

This section explores these concepts further and looks behind the drive to 'work together' as conformity and working together in a supportive climate. (supportive as perceived by the interviewees)

The need to 'fit in' (Melia, 1987) to the ward routine seemed to be the main motivational drive in the socialisation of nurses, and this is enacted in the interpersonal relationships between students and trained nurses on the ward. Certainly, the students' relationship with the ward staff seemed erratic and seemed driven by inclusion / exclusion issues. A process of self-stereotyping appears to occur which Turner, et. al., (1987) believed to be essential to conformity. The self-stereotyping takes the form of mentally associating with the group (any group, whether working or learning or leisure group) and internally taking on the attributes and norms which they see as belonging to the group. The notion of students going through many changes in self-stereotyping with every new (ward) group they work with over short periods of time conjures up images of a high degree of mental energy being directed towards knowing and keeping the ward group rules to maintain their social identity (op., cit.,). What can happen when a new group member brings rules into a working group can be gleaned by the following student's account.

This student was part of a new mature student group who were doing a more flexible training programme using continuous assessment strategies in line with a more self-directed curriculum. She found that there was a `them and us situation', with her tutor supporting her continuous assessment and resistance among the ward staff to take on the new assessment procedure from the School of Nursing, despite in-service training in the methods, because they saw them as time consuming. In an attempt to create a picture of students working together and working with trained staff in a supportive or non-supportive environment, I have chosen to reproduce an extensive account of this student's interview. I believe it illuminates well some of the underlying psychosocial processes in student / staff nurse interpersonal relationships. While exploring `the supportive environment' during the interview, I asked the student:

> JG: What does being supported mean to you?
>
> Student: I think it's being there, and listening to what you have to say, not necessarily agreeing with every word you say, but being there to listen... Like a friendly word... "How are you?" "Are you ok?" Just being there and to have a reasonably open relationship with someone. So you don't feel- what's the word? You must feel "psychologically safe", which I do with my tutor.. which makes a change sometimes from what you're having to deal with... on the ward.
>
> JG: So, is the ward situation sometimes psychologically unsafe for you?
>
> Student: Mm, sometimes....

She goes on to say:

> Not very often I must admit.. but.. the way we are treated as students, the hierarchy involved within nursing, it's sometimes quite acute and it is very difficult to communicate with people just on a reasonable level, because the hierarchy gets in the way. On the other hand it depends on where you go, because everywhere seems to be totally different in their way, looking at the way students are treated and the way staff nurses are treated... junior members of the ward team. But it is nice to have somewhere to go, if there

is a real problem, the tutor, I mean. I'm finding that I'm dealing with these problems now, whereas in my first year I wasn't.

JG: Right, So, when you say there's a hierarchy that makes it quite difficult to communicate even at a reasonable level, who are the people who constitute the hierarchy?

Student: At what level?

JG: Yes

Student: I don't think it is any one particular place...Sister and senior staff nurses, really.. and its sort of been explained because they are of the old school, so you just sort of put up with it. Since I've worked outside, (of nursing) and worked within, (nursing) obviously there are hierarchies there, you don't put up with it outside, if you see what I mean.

JG: Yes, so if you were in industry or in an office outside of nursing you would not experience the hierarchy in this way...?

Student: No..I don't think it exists... the hierarchical control I mean.. within a working framework, (outside of nursing) there tends to be more co-operation, and what is it, management by consensus...whereas in this particular field of nursing, (general nursing) it tends to be, you know,.. 'the buck stops here'. Which maybe it's a different way of looking at things. It's a different sort of work, so maybe that's why it's evolved as it has done. But you can go to other wards and your opinion is valued and you feel almost immediately part of the ward team and things tend to go from good to better, on Elderly Care and Mental Health, whereas there tends to be in some areas, stumbling blocks, between getting the work done, and doing the job that I'm supposed to be doing, which is learning as much as I can, plus obviously being part of the ward team and a pair of hands as well. I find that my attitude towards any sort of area of nursing is influenced really strongly by the people who actually work in those areas,. as well as the patients you are dealing with.

The tension this student is expressing can be illustrated thus:

186

Figure 6.3 Tension between personal needs, environmental support and work ethos

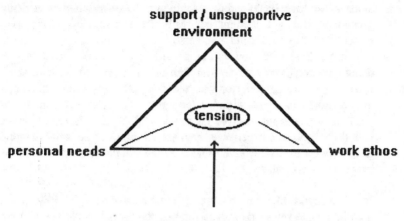

support / unsupportive
environment

tension

personal needs   work ethos

Creative / uncreative tension?

The angle of the pyramid which is dominant at ward level will affect how nurses perceive themselves to be psychologically safe or whether they will fear retribution. For example, if the work ethos in the form of oppressive hierarchical control is dominant this will strongly influence whether the student will even attempt to express personal needs for fear of retaliation, whereas if the work ethos is controlling yet supportive of patients' needs this will encourage students to believe that their needs will also be met. If the ward culture strongly supports the personal needs of students and / or encourages a supportive environment generally then students seem more able to express their needs with less fear of retribution.

In the above interview, the discussion went on to look at what this student needed from ward staff to have her learning needs met and still feel part of the working team, that is, still feel she was `pulling her weight'. Her main response was to return to her social needs again:

> If you said "good morning" to them in the morning, and when you've said "good morning" somebody replies ...just those sort of little things.

> JG: So it is actually being recognised as another human being?

> Student: Yes, I was talking to one of my classmates, and he said that he wasn't sure it was a good management tool to avoid eye contact all the time, you know, you walk into a room, this sort of thing, which I find extremely petty and annoying, and I'm not sure what the point is.

JG: Right, and you've had people who just don't make eye contact with you?

Student: No, (they don't) and if you chip in on a conversation, it suddenly goes silent, that sort of thing, but really, it's a recognition of you as a person, and it's you as quite a vulnerable sort of person as well. Because most of the time, when you start on a ward, you don't know what you are doing, you don't know where everything is, and you are not sure about what you should be doing or who you should be answerable to. But it usually works itself out within a fortnight, and you've got settled, and you're in a good team, and you get to know people and they get to know you. It can be a nice experience, even something as emotionally draining as Elderly Care... You tend to be able to draw the positive side of it to the people you work with.

JG: So it sounds like there needs to be quite a lot of dialogue between you and the people you work with in the first few weeks, while you sort out how this place works, and what your part is. What skills do the trained nurses need to help make you feel welcome, you've said the eye contact and just the `hellos', is there more that they can do if they are going to help you survive emotionally draining experiences?

Student: Things like just showing an interest, really, because I show an interest. I tend to sort of get in there both feet, read books. I tend to be a bit nosey, I like them to, maybe not show so much interest, but show an interest in my wellbeing, because I like to think that I show an interest in theirs.

The student repeated that people can demonstrate an interest by social enquiry, `how they are', `how the shift went', asking `what work needs doing', and goes on to say:

Student: Just trying to be part of the team, but you can only be part of the team if somebody wants you to be part of that team, and if you try and try and try, and all your getting is negativity back, maybe from just one or two people, but you know within the first two or three weeks, you know who you don't want to be on the shift with... mind you, maybe they think the same thing about me, you know! Really, to sort of meet half way..and so on..

JG: Why is it important for you to feel part of the team, to feel recognised by others?

Student: I think it's, well, it's one of the things that we have to do on our assessment sheet.

There is an educational obligation to get on well with the team, and the student will be assessed by her mentor and Ward Sister about her ability to work in the ward team.

JG: ..and to you as a person?

Student: I like to be liked. I like to have an opportunity for a social chit-chat.... I think it is just a basic need for me, you know, to be friendly with people, and I suppose thereby to be part of the gang. It's difficult for me to be on the outside. I don't like being.. I don't mind being the new girl, because being the new girl doesn't last very long .. and then you become part of things, and you, yes, I think, I always gain so much from an experience if I am part of the team and I can relate well with people that I am with. I tend to get very negative and moody I suppose, if my efforts to be part of the team aren't recognised, or thought less of, or sometimes, not very often, but sometimes it's "Oh God, a student" you know...It doesn't happen very often.

JG: What happens to you when it does?

Student: I get cross

JG: Because?

Student: Because I think it's thoughtless

JG: Mme..

Student: ..and I think they ought to have a refresher course on being a student

JG: What would that do?

Student: If they went to a new ward and somebody said, "Oh golly, it's the new staff nurse, she doesn't know anything!" I wonder how it would make her feel, but it makes me cross. It used to upset me, but it just makes me cross now, because I don't think they should be in a position of authority.

JG: You said earlier that it is not so bad now, in your second year, because you were managing to deal with some of these things yourself, whereas in the first year, you did rely more on the tutors. How are you dealing with them?

Student: I'm being more assertive, really.

JG: Can you say more?

Student: I tend to point things out to people. Not very often, but, I don't know...

And the student goes on to recount the problems she had in getting co-operation from the trained staff to fill in her assessment forms. It is essential for the student to document the nursing experiences on the assessment form, and the trained staff are obliged to assess the standards of her work and grade her. If the documentation is not done correctly the student can be referred. When she pointed this out to her mentor on one ward, she was told "to put them away and forget about them until the end.." (of the ward experience). The student went on:

> Well, it has to be filled in. I have to have a half-way interview and I have to have a final interview and the final interview has to be two weeks before we finish the ward allocation, so should I not be able to cover any of the standards by then, I can cover them in the last two weeks, and if I don't do it, I'll be referred. And she said, the mentor "Don't worry about it, don't worry about it, you'll pass with flying colours"..

The student then had to make the staff nurse aware that the tutor would be monitoring the process, she also referred to the ultimate authority of the ENB (English National Board, who have a statutory right to approve courses in nursing) to support her need to have her assessments done correctly and on time and to convince the staff nurse to comply with her needs. As she said:

> I don't like being in the position where the School is telling me one thing, which I believe is perfectly reasonable, and the ward is saying another, which to me is unreasonable, and of course we, students, are stuck in the middle....and we are not getting any back-up from the ward.

The above extended account highlights this student's confusion about how different wards function under different social codes of practice when relating to student nurses and even to junior trained nurses on the ward. This student saw a difference in social norms between nursing staff on Psychiatric and Care of the Elderly wards and social norms among staff on some general medical, surgical and other specialist wards. She recognised that very hierarchical relations blocked communication

190

which she found detrimental as 'she needed to feel psychologically safe..' which for her meant; to be listened to; to be part of the social fabric on the ward; to be liked and respected which, when it did not happen, interfered with her learning as a student. She compared the Psychiatric and Care of the Elderly wards against others saying that in the former she felt her opinions were valued and that she was helped to feel effective as a team member very quickly. In a previous section of this chapter these two clinical areas of nursing were described as less technical with more emphasis placed on nursing care which could be custodial or psychosocial caring. However, as I said then, from my observations on the ward, I believe that the emphasis on which type of care is given is more a matter of the ward culture than the medical specialism, and this is particularly so when it comes to how nurses support and care for each other. This assertion is based on the finding in this study that students found some Psychiatric and Care of the Elderly wards more custodial and regimental rather than social caring and patient-orientated.

For this student, positive experiences in some wards allowed her to accept that she was capable of working in a team and capable of 'fitting in' to new wards relatively easily, but that this depended very much on the ward culture. She also compared different working relationships within nursing with other work experience she had as a team member in a managerial position in a large Company before she started nurse training. Her comparisons of the different cultures reflected poorly on how nurses structured their work and their relationships. Her tutor gave her a reason for the hierarchical structure and way of behaving in some wards, by saying that the senior staff were of 'the old School' which implies that although their behaviour was inappropriate, there was little to be done about it. Somehow the explanation had to suffice to help the students 'put up with it.' This acceptance of the insolubility of problems offered to the students by the tutors occurred a number of times. It has an undertone of encouraging helplessness in the new entrants to the organisational culture and is contrary to Harré (1983) definition of personal agency which means to conceive oneself as capable of operating from a place of ultimate power of decision and action in relation to oneself.

This student's account mirrors those of most of the ward staff interviewed. A third year student nurse summarised what she meant be support on the ward by listing:

> ..time for people to listen to me; verbally supporting me; recognising I am
> a human being with my weaknesses and limitations and where possible to
> change working practices when it gets too heavy.. that is, to lighten your
> load.

There is a richness in these accounts about students' entry into new wards; about the skills they need to enable them to negotiate their learning needs which seem to be in direct competition for trained staff's time with ward work and patients care and about the students' need to inform trained staff regarding the educational obligations they have and how they are to be met. This educational need included the need for trained staff to provide opportunities for learners to experience team work so they can be assessed on their ability to work in a team. The need this student had for social recognition mirrors the need the patients have for social and emotional recognition and interaction (Smith, 1992). This highlights the concept of the collective unconscious psychosocial agenda which all individuals bring to relationships, that is, the need for recognition, (Berne, 1961) upon which appeasement of that agenda, relationships stand or fall. It makes foreground my tentative hypothesis *that the psychosocial caring imperative needs to permeate the whole working world of nurses so that they can be therapeutic agents for themselves as well as their patients*. This was the opinion of one tutor, and was echoed by many:

> I agree strongly that nurses need to be able to support each other if they are to be enabling to patients.

The above account and those of others in this research can be set alongside a functional empowerment model being developed by Roberts (1993) for the purpose of assessing both the personal experience and the organisational culture which creates such experiences. This model reflects a hierarchy of personal needs which empowers individuals to be effective at a work group and organisational level, where:

> Self-empowerment is a process by which one increasingly takes greater charge of oneself and one's life. By (our) definition it is not an end-state. One cannot become a `self-empowered person'. It is a process of becoming in which one behaves in a more or less empowered way. (Hopson & Scally, 1981, p.57)

Figure 6.4 Functional empowerment cycle

Celebration
effective functioning
good communication

positive relations
(spiritual - physical)

\ /
safety
/ \

(emotional - intellectual)

This is an up-hierarchy, with safety needs being the first priority before any other attribute can operate effectively. Safety needs are met and continuously nurtured by:

Having a positive regard for the other

acceptance of self and others

praise for work done.

(Roberts 1993)

Such nurturing attributes were found to be important in this study and supports Firth, et. al., (1986) findings regarding interpersonal support amongst nurses at work. It also supports the buberian concept of the need to begin interacting with others from an 'I-thou' relationship (Buber, 1937) where we value who we are as human beings as a necessary first step to creating a sense of safety. (see Chapter 1)

In Roberts' model, safety as 'psychological safety' is very like the student's account in this section: of being recognised; being listened to; being respected and being valued for who she is and for her contributions to patient care and team effort. It also embraces Cherniss' (1980) description of support, that is: feedback on performance; information, advice or technical assistance; and emotional support or ventilation of feelings.

The emphasis here is that safety needs must be operating at an effective level for nurses to want to have positive relations with others. If nurses, like any work group, are not feeling psychologically secure then their behaviour becomes self-protective; with-holding and unco-operative. From positive relations, people will invest time

193

and energy in developing good communications between individuals and the whole team. From here the springboard into effective functioning at the group and organisational level takes off with celebration for achievements as a necessary and natural follow-through. This celebration will feed back into creating more safety, more security. The hallmark of such a culture is spontaneity, creativity and honest communication. The consequence of lack of safety for group and organisational functioning can be illustrate by a downhill spiral.

Figure 6.5 The dysfunctional (dis-empowerment) cycle

(spiritual - physical)

No Safety

(emotional -intellectual)

Negative interpersonal relations

poor communication

ineffective functioning

conflict, hassles, violence.

The factors which feed this negative cycle are

blaming behaviour

humiliation

disregarding at the level of being.

(Roberts 1993)

Examples of such dysfunctional behaviour within work groups is evident to a degree in this research. Evidence such as:

> No personal confrontation should be done in front of patients. They, (the trained staff) should respect your feelings and not stand lecturing you in the middle of the ward. (student)

And from a junior staff nurse:

...and I just couldn't stand it any more, being abused in front of people, in front of patients and doctors.. being shouted at and one thing and another.. just feeling like, why am I here, there is no reason for me to be here... not doing anything valuable..

This staff nurse spoke to the senior staff nurse with whom she had found it difficult to work and asked that they try to resolve their differences. The senior staff nurse's response was to:

Hit the roof, she went absolutely mad, screaming and shouting. I was really upset, and crying and the patients noticed, and I went out to the balcony and stayed out there for a while. (Staff Nurse)

Firth, et. al., (1986) study of interpersonal support from superiors to nurses at work, (in psychiatric and mental handicap settings-as they were then called) came up with similar findings which was that trained nurses perceived themselves to be in a supportive environment when they experienced 'a non-possessive warmth or respect, accurate empathy and genuineness or emotional openness.' (Rogerian (1967) concepts of an enabling relationship). This seems to be the cry of the students in general hospitals too.

The first student's account in this section demonstrated that she managed the group dynamics in the ward better in the second year as she was more assertive in 'pointing things out to people'. Here, we see that assertiveness, one of the interpersonal skills listed in the S.O.N.(1) curriculum, when used by students for their own benefit can ease their passage through the various wards.

Other interviewees' comments of a supportive working environment confirmed Cherniss' (1980) descriptions with the definition spanning from being therapeutic to patients to working together with a common philosophy and nursing goals. From the account given by the student Andy receiving feedback on performance was not forthcoming, nor the emotional support offered which was needed in cases of difficulty, personal or work related. I asked one tutor:

JG: So what happens when the students experience traumatic events?

Tutor: Students may get support from the senior staff if they have just been through a recognised traumatic event, like a cardiac arrest or a death, but most of the time they have to overtly show they are in need by crying.. before they are offered any support.

And for another nurse tutor working with a student on the ward, her idea of support was:

Supporting comes in what we say afterwards, when you have dealt with the nursing situation, "Now.. what about us, we need to be honest with each other and talk things over".

This tutor would then give feedback and evaluate the student's performance in a way she perceived as supportive. One student's definition of 'therapeutic' included the concept of teamwork. In this study the wish to accept the student's phenomenological worldview allows one to accept the possibility that working with team spirit can be a healing process for nurses. As she said:

Therapeutic means balancing things out and working as a team. The team, that you should help each other individually, the environment should be therapeutic.

Here the team is seen to be responsible for creating the therapeutic environment. A tutor supported this by saying:

I think they should be able to work together, as a team. We all have a philosophy of our nursing, what we think nursing is, that we incorporate into our practice.

and therefore:

Nurses should work together, same philosophy, same language, similar concepts.

And yet:

People who manage to work on their own don't want to get involved with others problems. It's enough work to look after yourself. There is no energy for others, or they are just not interested. There is no team spirit. (Student)

and:

Generally people working on the ward get on well with each other, they have to or else there won't be any unity and the nursing care falls apart. (Staff Nurse)

But for another tutor:

Nurses are not enabling for each other. They do not support each other on a psychological level even if they support each other as a team on a practical level.

This confusion of different perspectives highlights the kaleidoscope of experiences that nurses can have on different wards and which they need to take account of if they are to adapt to the ward culture.

For Andy, the student, team work was more like the definition of the work group mentioned earlier, that is: "Minimum interaction among staff, no personal issues, get on with the job", all of which could have been an acceptance of ward norms, (and could have been a carry-over from family and previous educational experience as a pattern of working in hierarchical ways), and it certainly did not allow for emotional support or the ventilation of feelings.

A third year student who was very stressed declared that:

> How am I being cared for?.. *(long pause..)* I don't feel there are a lot of wards where you do feel cared for. You feel used most of the time, by the senior staff, they use you, definitely. A lot of them, not all of them, act as if students can carry on regardless, like robots. I've been on many wards where a lot of senior staff are like that. It's very rare to get good support as a student. I don't know what it is like for trained staff, but for students there is no support.

The attributes needed to create a supportive environment include respect for the individual and skills in interpersonal relating which are enabling. Most participants in this study felt they lacked the confidence to be supportive to peers in the same way they were expected to be supportive to patients. One needs to know more about the relationship between nurses to find out why they do not, in their view, receive or give support spontaneously, and what other concepts operate to force nurses to conform to belong to the ward team, even when they are not happy to do so. According to one Staff Nurse:

> We need to recognise our attitudes, be self-aware, to be supportive of others.

For this Staff Nurse understanding her personal beliefs and values which directed her behaviour was an important step to being supportive to others.

It proved difficult to separate out the various contexts in which interviewees thought they were un-supported. There seemed to be a lot of pessimism on the wards regarding support, that is, nurses were either left alone to get on with the work, or avoided if 'things' were not going smoothly. The working relationships seemed emotionally distant, and it seemed harder to 'practise' enabling skills with peers who were not 'technically ill'. Yet, this was contradicted by one tutor's account:

> As a Ward Sister, I was a patient, and the students I knew kept away from me. I suppose they found me threatening. In the end I gave up asking for anything, pain relief, drinks. I was isolated in my cubicle for days.

This tutor concluded that:

> Nurses don't treat their colleagues well when they become patients. I guess it is a fear of doing something wrong and being found out and criticised.

My impression was that nurses avoid that level of intimacy (interpersonalising according to Beverley (1988)) for fear that:

(1)   Peers might reject them (whereas patients cannot reject them so easily)

(2)   Peers might give the helper negative feedback, which might undermine the helper's perceptions of how effective they are with patients. Patients tend not to give nurses direct negative feedback on their interpersonal skills.

Nurses seemed to have problems sharing interpersonal expertise with each other for example, counselling or enabling skills. There seemed to be a confusion of role boundaries, that is, nurses are nurses, not patients, so should not need `nursing' which then gets translated into nurses should not need psychosocial support.

It is in the nature of a grounded theory study that when asking individuals what their perceptions are of a phenomenon, their account will be idiosyncratic. Each person will speak from their own core needs which will influence their selective interpretation of events to address these needs. The nature of the basic sociopsychological process in any research is a recognition of how the individual and the group balances the intrapersonal and the interpersonal processes, which is a problem (as a challenge) in group dynamic terms. Hence asking nurses how they perceive they are supported at work will raise significant differences in answers about expectations and interpretations. What was salient as a category in this research was that most participants stated that emotional support and being recognised and valued as a human being was very important and absent to a large extent.

A summary of teamwork is offered as it developed from theoretical memoing.

♦   Team work is about "getting the work done" with the minimum interaction between nurses or engaging in personal agenda.

♦   Personal distance is valued and sought by nurses preferring to work alone where possible.

♦   There seemed to be many `shoulds' and `oughts' about splitting the personal from `professional' work under the guise of professionalism. Bringing in personal content was seen as an inferior way of working. `It could impinge' on your work.

198

♦   Hiding real feelings was considered 'appropriate' behaviour.

♦   Being dishonest to patients was legitimate to keep them happy.

Yet there was a strong belief that co-operation among nurses was very important as it kept the nursing care intact, that is 'not falling apart'. Managing the interface between personal needs, the interpersonal relationship and the professional nature of nurses working as a team seems a potent area to engage in for the purpose of creating an enabling environment.

Many of the above issues link the category 'Conforming to try to belong to the ward team' with the category 'Professional shield' which will be discussed later in this chapter.

The concepts which reflected most obviously the elements of the supportive environment are shown below:

Indicators of the concept: Supporting each other (The 'wished for' dimension)

- respecting others' point of view
- making time to talk through distressing events with senior staff or peers
- sympathy and understanding-for trust building, for people to disclose
- quality of caring implies interest in person, that is, internal quality of caring
- going beyond social conversation.
- respecting individuality and acknowledging uniqueness
- recognising personal strengths and building from strengths
- self-awareness implies potential to develop personal attributes to be enabling for others

These indicators of the concept 'Supporting each other' on the ward are similar to the indicators of the concept 'Belonging in the learning set' discussed in Chapter 4. This would seem obvious as the issue is one of 'belonging' with 'supporting' as a co-variant to 'belonging'. The 'wished for' dimension in brackets above gives a sense of the tone in which most participants spoke of being supported. All had some experience within nursing, and before starting nursing, of what 'belonging' and social / emotional support' meant, some sharing this experience particularly from the Psychiatric and Care of the Elderly placements. The conclusion is that whether nurses feel they 'belong' or are 'supported' depends on others already in the ward team, so the locus of control is external to them which creates the helplessness (Seligman, 1975) experienced in their interpersonal relationships. This was well illustrated by a student in response to my question:

> JG: So you take risks, to challenge an unfair ward report, so that you don't undermine your self-confidence?

Student: I've got to, but actually, I've been seeing a Counsellor since last year...

JG: So that has helped?

Student: That has helped, because I think last time I saw you, I had done my exams, I walked out... I had to go back and do it, because I was really- that's nursing for you, It certainly doesn't help your confidence, because since I've been nursing, I've definitely lost my confidence.

JG: What does nursing do? Where does this happen?

Student: I think it undermines. I think this staffing bit... it's not the patients, it's the people that you work with, a real problem. I think if you asked anyone in our set, they would say exactly the same thing, there is no real problem with the work you do, with the patients, the problem is with the staff. If you get on, fine. If someone doesn't like you you're really in trouble, because you find that they are bitchy, they can undermine you, they can make your life absolutely hell on the ward- or they can make it really pleasant. And I think, I just wasn't used to that.. and I mean, I don't think you find that sort of pressure, the way you're treated, anywhere else, in offices, in ..oppression is a good word for it.

This last statement indicates just how tense relationships can get and the effect it can have on the individual. The tension illustrated in Figure 6.6 can be shown on a dimensional scale.

Figure 6.6   The dimensions of factors which create tension in conforming
to try to belong to the ward team

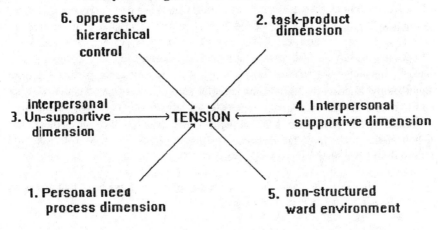

Some of the categories above, the hierarchical dimension, (6) and the un-supportive / competitive environment (3) have strong links with the category 'present a united front' (see Figure 6.1,) and managing the interface between respecting hierarchical 'expert' authority, hierarchical control, their silence about poor standards of care and the competitive environment in the wards which will be discussed under the core category 'Professional shield' in the next section.

However, before leaving this section it is worth noting that many of the issues in this section on teamwork focused mainly on the social psychological process of inclusion / exclusion, expressed as a need to belong and be supported rather than on teamwork as defined in earlier in this chapter. This is an important distinction to be made as the issues surrounding inclusion / exclusion in groups makes understandable why nurses will conform and will keep silent about poor standards of care and about expressing their own needs. Taking on a Moscovici strategy for change as a lone dissenter in a group has been proven to be ineffective (Moscovici & Lage, 1976). The student, by virtue of the short periods of time spent on each ward, coupled with her/ his student status has a particularly hazardous route to navigate through the different training wards, especially where reprisals are possible in terms of bad ward reports if she or he mis-judges the norms or mood of the ward culture.

The professional shield

While the section on 'Conform to try to belong to the ward team' focused more inwardly on how individuals understood the role of conforming in relation to working on the wards, that is, working fast and working as a team, this section looks more at the outward face which nurses showed by way of main strategies they used to accommodate to the ward culture and the hospital nursing culture generally. This explanation will be done through exploring the sub-categories under the core category 'The professional shield'.

Presenting a united front

The need to present a united front was an agreed norm endorsed by many ward nurses, students, and tutors, which influenced the nurse-nurse relationship significantly. It meant that disagreements between nurses were not spoken of on the ward; nurses remained cheerful regardless of how they felt, which was well expressed by one staff nurse, Kate and will be discussed in the next section. The notion of the professional facade sprang to mind early in the fieldwork and was followed up when appropriate. The professional facade for 'patients' sake', took the form of:

You have to make it look as though you get on well together on the wards to try to keep the patients happy. Patients will get worried if they see nurses unhappy or disagreeing. Nurses will be seen as weak and not coping.

And the same student:

If the trained staff have some gripe against you, not of a working nature, but personal, they should not deal with it on the 'shop floor'. Nurses have a professional aspect of their work, they also have personal aspects which might impinge on the professional. You have two lives really, the personal and professional, you should never mix them up.

The above statements show sensitive awareness of personal aspects of work which would seem on the surface to be acceptable professional practice, however, what often lay behind such statements was that nurses found it difficult to express their real thinking and feelings and that suppression was rewarded by being called 'professional practice'.

The perceived fear was that patients, who, according to one student, "had little else to do but observe nurses working", would be looking out for any sign of weaknesses or conflict among nurses and feed their anxiety on that. According to one tutor:

As a patient, it would not help me if a nurse broke down in front of me, bursting into tears, because I am the one who is dying. Patients need somebody strong to lean on.

The purpose of the professional facade is to prevent patients worrying so that they will trust that the nurses know what they are doing and that they are in control. This 'knowing what is going on' was a front according to some students and junior staff nurses, who confessed to pretending at times that they knew patients diagnoses, problems and treatment to 'reassure the patient'. Much of this aspect of the nurse-patient relationship is not part of this study; however the 'professional mask' is a cultural phenomenon learnt by nurses from each other on the wards and as such is an important part of how nurses relate to each other.

Another example of professional facade is how nurses manage the complexity of 'acting professionally' and strategies they use to deal with the standards of (clinical) care given to patients. One tutor's comment was:

Junior staff have more difficulty in maintaining high standards, pressure of work, for one. A lot of people nursing by the bedside are in a situation where they are actually not meeting the standards they would like to meet. Those nurses who make a noise (complain) about not being able to maintain good standards and trying to do something about it, are being professional. But those who say "Oh well, there's nothing we can do about it" are the ones who are being un-professional. Nurses who get tired of trying to improve things must have a difficult time. I know that for myself, If I was in that position, I wouldn't actually be able to stay in the job. That to me is being professional.

JG: What does it mean to be professional?

Tutor: To me, being professional is looking at and trying to clearly decide for myself what I think and feel on certain issues, and set standards that I see as necessary, standards of behaviour, of dress, appropriate to the role. Being professional means sticking to those standards, in the sense that I'm prepared to put my neck on the line for something I believe in, but not doing it in an aggressive manner, but doing it in an appropriate manner.

The tutor went on to say that although she would like to be flexible and see other nurses' point of view, she will stand up for what she thinks is right, and will not be told how she should think on clinical issues. A student nurse was quite distressed when talking of standards of nursing care and interpersonal conflict:

Nurses are often reluctant to say 'poor standards of care' given to patients by colleagues. Insufficient staffing levels is the rationalisation given... in reality... they are frightened of having the cards marked, so to speak.

The above accounts indicate that maintenance of standards of care has an interpersonal dimension among nurses as well as affecting patient care. To 'be professional', one would need to condemn poor clinical practice when it occurs, yet who is to be condemned? How one would condemn another and what the consequences are of speaking out, are important issues. Nurses are obliged to stay on the ward regardless of standards, without industrial action, or reporting serious incidents to the general public. The alternatives are to stay in nursing and be silent or get out. A recent report on 'Maladministration and redress' (HMSO 1993/4) has recommended that nurses be free to express their concern about standards of care with the health service commissioner. Whichever way this recommendation goes, in this study nurses experienced conflict between wanting to nurse to a high standard and not being able to do so. This situation forces people to make decision about whether they will stay in nursing or not. The interpersonal skills needed to confront another person in an enabling way are part of the skills of assertiveness which is advocated as part of the interpersonal skills training in the School of Nursing. Yet nurses do not seem to know how to use such skills. Without the skills of confronting constructively or because of fear of the consequences of confrontation nurses seem to be limited to either silence or leaving nursing. (Moores & Thompson, 1975 and Lindop, 1989) The problem of being silent is that you can get ill, if the silence is the suppression of emotions. In Chapter 1, Heron's (1992) definition of emotional competence included the ability for people to be aware of issues which cause them distress capable to manage situations in an emotionally healthy way. As Heron states:

> So old hurt-laden agendas are not projected, nor transferred, into current situations. It means being able to spot institutionalised and professional forms of displacement, and to find ways of replacing them with more rational, flexible and adaptive behaviour. (Heron, 1992, p.131)

However, distressed silence is seen every day in hospitals, as one tutor put it:

> People (nurses) often come to the levels where they are having more sickness-due to stress-yet managers won't automatically think, maybe that person needs more support. No, you have to really break down and cry and say 'I can't cope' otherwise people won't see. They don't look at each others faces enough to know how they feel.

It would be difficult for managers to act on the knowledge that students or staff nurses are too physically and emotionally stressed, as they would then be faced with the problem of who would do the work if nurses are allowed to go off sick or for a rest. When the Salmon Report (HMSO 1966) was implemented and nurses managed nurses, it was easier to hire temporary nurses through an external agency to cover sickness, holidays and so on. That is unlikely to happen in the present managerial and economic environment of strict non-nursing financial control of staffing numbers on the wards. During this study, students were an essential part of the work force, rather than supernumerary, so they were under pressure to be both workers and learners. But notice that the options seem limited, to be either supernumerary, or take time off sick rather than support-while-remaining in-work. How this might be remedied will be discussed in Chapter 7.

The most striking evidence of lack of nurturing in an organism is when it feels so deprived it becomes sick.

> Nursing causes physical stress, much time off sick is deliberate time out rather than time sick. (Tutor)

And another tutor:

> Students need to be protective of self.. only expose themselves to as much patient contact as they can manage.. I see a lot of nurses coping strategies, on duty and off: the degree of avoidance, the unpopular patient, the patient whom they feel uncomfortable with, so patients don't get much attention.

And yet another tutor:

Some nurses are stressed and avoid difficult situations by shuffling papers in the office-to avoid situations like crying and distressed patients.

What are the main stressors for nurses on the ward? Are they related to the illnesses of the patients and the demands that are put on them, or are they the relationships the nurses have on the ward, with both patients and staff? Guppy (1991) found that the two main factors causing stress in nurses were (1) interpersonal relations and resource problems and (2) dealing with death. The findings in this study indicate that the interpersonal relationships are the tensions which can cause most stress to nurses. According to Rabkin & Struening, (1976) the link between stressful events and illness is typically very small. It has become more illuminative to look at `resistance resources' to make sense of why many people lead what could be stressful lives and remain well. It seems useful to state here what are the attributes which help individuals stay well under stress as these are attributes which can be taught as part of personal and interpersonal skills training. The main attributes have been found to be "interpersonal relational resources" (Antonovsky, 1979, p.114) which have been conceptualised as;

- receiving direct assistance from some others,
- affirmation of one's beliefs and practices from a group,
- being liked by significant others,
- and knowing a lot of people who all know each other (Kobasa, 1982, pp.168-177)

This can be seen as approximating the functional empowerment cycle (Figure 6.4) particularly addressing psychological safety and how it could create positive relations, leading to effective communication. The qualities needed for psychological safety are the same: being valued, being part of a supportive group, having enabling assistance and receiving feedback in the form of affirmations which all help reduce un-productive stress and could instead create a stimulating productive learning environment.

> Nurses' communication skills and interpersonal skills are helping nurses
> with the stress of patients unburdening their problems.. you see very sad
> things going on and if they know all the psychological processes, they have
> all this self-awareness, perhaps it can help them sort out their own feelings
> as well as empathising with patients. (Tutor)

Antonovsky's (1979) concepts take on a psychological and interpersonal perspective to stress resistance, which fits with the notion of psychological safety. If one looked at some of the benefits for nurses of learning interpersonal skills, then resistance to stress induced illness in the form of positive interpersonal relational resources would be significant. Lutzen (1990) found that psychiatric nurses managed to reduce tension brought about by moral sensing and ideological conflict by seeking emotional support from peers. Nurses within the general hospitals could also benefit by being more emotionally supportive to each other.

To return to the concept of silence, one student's account reflected what many others said, which was:

> People working together as peers are not being open and sharing what they feel about things, about what they see is wrong, it's avoiding conflict.

There is collusive silence about poor standards of nursing care. Some of the reasons are that nurses avoid conflict (see later in this chapter) when it comes to clinical practice and they will not support a peer speaking out, another is that when the permanent staff are content with their standards of nursing care, they are resentful of being told that the nursing practice is poor, particularly if told by students. In one incident:

> Support is stronger than caring. Support is when people will back you up, stand up for you. Recently a consultant wanted to put eusol on a women's leg wound, but the product has been banned and withdrawn. I tried to tell the consultant; `I'm sorry, we haven't got this...' I was not allowed to finish the sentence... I was ordered to do it. The person in charge who was junior (junior staff nurse) just said `yes'. So where is our professionalism if we are going to keep being intimidated like this. I would have like the full backing of the staff to say no to the consultant.

> JG: Do you think you would get it?

> Student: No, because people are too frightened of consultants, the nursing staff, I mean, fear of getting into trouble, being on a disciplinary charge. The problem is that there is often a lack of maturity, lack of assertiveness and conviction in the knowledge we have.

Issues of silence can be summarised thus:

- fear of reprisal
- absence of unity between colleagues (despite the need to have a united front for patients)
- lack of skills in confronting poor standards (or)
- fear to confront, that is, fear of conflict

As Beardshaw (1981) stated, silence is a normal human response to intimidation and fear.

In Chapter 5 when discussing assertiveness skills the notion of teaching assertiveness too early was highlighted. The message seemed to be not to train people in the skills of speaking out until they had been on the ward long enough to understand the clinical specialism, and understand the ward routine. For the students, their need to speak out concerned basic social and hygiene care for patients and about how they themselves were treated. As the students spent between six to twelve weeks on average in a ward, their knowledge of the specialism would probably never be robust enough to challenge that, however, general care, psychosocial care and their experience of how the felt they 'belong' and 'supported' begins the first time they walk onto a ward or even into the School of Nursing.

Did the tutors' behaviour mirror the impotence of students on the ward to make changes or to break their silence? Tutors can be seen as good role models of powerlessness about standards of nursing on wards when they will not confront poor standards themselves. One tutor reasoned:

> Who am I really, I am just another interfering nosey person from the School, telling the staff what they should do.

And later in the interview:

> I find it difficult to confront trained staff. We tutors carry the flag for the School and they see us as interfering. When the boat is rocked between the Service side and the School it is really rocked. Then they don't want you on the ward. They tend not to want to co-operate and probably talk about the School to the students. There is a certain lack of loyalty.

The tutor speaking about professionalism reflected the saying that ideal people end up teaching rather than practising. Leaving nursing rather than practising seems a poor option, especially if one trains others to nurse. Can tutors justify training people to nurse in a way that is not practicable?

If nurses find it difficult to maintain high standards, could that be one of the reasons for the hierarchy, that is, distancing from patients, as the more you know how you should nurse, and the more you find it difficult to apply this knowledge in practice, the more you might distance yourself to protect self from the sense of helplessness. Marshall (1980) found that emotional detachment and denial of feelings were the result of high stress amongst nurses. A sense of helplessness, that is, being unable to influence outcomes (Seligman 1975) will create emotional distancing, a concept which has similar characteristics to the core sociopsychological process of with-holding as a strategy for managing self found to operate in the School of Nursing. One trained counsellor who was also a nurse teacher said that most nurses wanting to train in counselling, realised that the hospital system was geared towards fast throughput with no time for the processes of nurturing which they saw as an essential part of nursing. This caused such nurses tremendous pain and propelled them into non-nursing therapeutic professions.

Although this research has focused on the personal and interpersonal relationship dimensions among nurses themselves, the importance of the organisational dimension cannot be ignored. In this study the organisational dimension has had its main impact on how nurses viewed nursing standards. Within an organisational culture, which seemed to encourage silence and conformity it is difficult to understand why nurses were asked to learn interpersonal skills. The art of leaving boundaries fuzzy (Graham 1981) with regards to which type of interpersonal relationships are acceptable and which are not is an issue of power and control which will be discussed in a later section of this chapter. One wonders if the interpersonal skills training advocated in the S.O.N.(1) was aimed at learning how to wear the professional mask or whether it was to move towards authenticity as is intended in humanistic education. Jourard (1971) believes that professional training encourages graduates to wear a professional mask, to limit their behaviour to the range that proclaims their professional status. A question in the early part of this research was who are the `mask makers'. I had a strong sense of this `mask developing' when nurses constantly referred to the teaching of interpersonal skills in experiential workshops as artificial and therefore unnecessary and a waste of time for them, and that the skills would come naturally to them when they were in uniform and with `real patients'. It seems that they would put on a mantle of an `enabling interpersonal relating' like putting on a smile as they go to a patient's bedside and put away their enabling intentions and behaviour as they move away from the bedside. This is not the nature of being a therapeutic agent in a caring environment, but rather the stress of wearing a professional mask to shield oneself from authentic emotional engagement with patients and colleagues.

Respecting authority and hierarchical control

There is a hierarchical status in nursing which brings with it respect, a valuing of opinion, of expertise as well as a distancing from direct physical care of patients. Junior nurses particularly acknowledge and are content with the notion of Schein's (1988) description of rational authority (expert power) and positional power (Paton, et. al., 1985) in their seniors.

Part of the problem for students is knowing how to influence nursing practice without seemingly having expert power. According to the staff, students have no right to influence ward policy or practice just because they are working on the ward. Influencing is allowed by those who are seen to be knowledgeable which is often defined in terms of seniority. That is, the person who has been here longest or has the higher rank will know best.

208

> People listen to intuition based on nursing experience, not on intuition
> without experience. (Student)

> When you are very junior you don't have the necessary knowledge and
> skills to support your argument to authority figures. A lot of support comes
> from knowledge. The fact that you can argue your case from facts and
> figures. (another Student).

An example was given of the valuing (or devaluing) of experience by two enrolled
nurses who were doing the two year `conversion' course to [9]Registered General
Nurse. They were allowed to help trained staff with the cardiac monitors as they had
both trained in Intensive Care nursing but could not help with policy decisions or
ward routines, even though they had been trained nurses on general wards for some
years.
Andy, (the first student), decided that trying to influence change was a waste of
time:

> Things need to change on the ward (practices), but when you talk about
> changing things at report, they might think, "You have only been here five
> minutes, you don't know nought". You have no hope of saying what you
> think, so you give up, and do what they tell you. It would be the best thing
> really. Do what you are told and get on with the work to the best of your
> ability.

> No hope of saying what you think about making ward management
> changes, as too junior. So you give up, do what you are told, go by the
> book without anyone getting hurt.

> JG: What do you mean by that?

> Andy: Don't show your feelings on the ward if you don't like the
> management, deal with them, your feelings, outside work.

The same `separating out' of nurses into student and non-student was experienced
by Post-Registration registered psychiatric nurse students whose skills in
interpersonal relating were seldom if ever valued or used by the trained nurses on
the wards. One student said that she puzzled a lot as to why trained nurses did not
find out from the students what life experience they brought to the ward, such as
being in a long term relationship, having children, having cared for dependents. She
went on to say:

209

Nobody gets to know each other, and in every other job that I have done, there's normally a social aspect to it, and there is no social aspect, and I think that is a shame. I must admit that once a couple of staff nurses knew I had children their attitude changes..

JG: In what way?

Especially when they found out their ages (her children were aged 17 and 19 years), they said, Oh, I thought you were under twenty-six years old...... They showed me more respect, which I think is bad, they should show the same respect to all students regardless of their age. It shouldn't make a difference.

There is certainly a problem in the interpersonal relationships about being valued or being ignored. Students and junior staff raised this issue continuously. What seemed to be valued was hierarchical status and the ability to influence ward decisions and even the ward culture. This may be one of the reasons why students say that they cannot wait to be promoted up the hierarchy, so that people will begin to take them seriously and listen to them.

So there may be appropriate hierarchy and deference given to knowledgeable people who know what is best for the patients, and when such legitimate authority, whether through expertise or managerial role is used constructively then junior staff accept it and learn from such experiences. However, there seemed to be very fuzzy boundaries between what was legitimate authority with proper use of that authority, and what was oppressive and inappropriate power-over others. This will be the subject of the next section. This section concludes with one tutor's assessment:

There is appropriate hierarchy ..We are all guided by the legal aspects of the profession. But it is back to self awareness, being aware that the way I like to do things isn't going to be the way that other people like to do things. What is important for me will not necessarily be important for somebody else.

When the category `support in ward based relationships' was isolated and developed over the interviews it interrelated with the notion of a united front, to feed into the category of `Conformity to try to belong to the ward team.' For such strategies to work for nurses without causing too much stress particularly the sense of helplessness; the need to distance themselves from actively engaging interpersonally was isolated. This category started as `professionalism' (see Chapter 3) or the correct way to behave at the descriptive level, and moved at a theoretical process level as `the professional facade'. Here it touched on nurses suppressing their thoughts and feelings for the patients' sake, but in the final synthesis of data became the

'Professional shield', as a strategy for managing helplessness / powerlessness articulated finally as:

> Fearing intimacy in the form of openness about self and honesty with others

in their working relationships.

This salient category of 'Professional shield' was recognised as a basic socio-psychological process with the recurring evidence that nurses talked of protecting themselves from the unsupportive nature of their interpersonal relationships and the exclusion experienced in staff working relationships. Elements of the category are given in abbreviated form below to show the interlinking robust nature of the core basic socio-psychological process.

Dimensions of the professional shield

Causes of professional shield:
¨   Fear of put-down
¨   fear of rejection
¨   supportive / caring skills are up for scrutiny by peers and senior nurses
¨   Inability to support psychologically

Figure 6.7 Characteristics of the professional shield

Characteristics of "The professional shield": Further indicators of the category:	Psychological processes: Distancing:
• Professional implies loss of personal identity • Uniform helps here-we hide behind it • Smile, make believe we are happy for the patients' sake • Teams are about tasks, not emotional support • Too busy (with tasks) to care about patients or other nurses • Silence about poor standards of care for patients' sake. Links with belonging / not belonging to ward team	Focus is on 'getting it right' as "professional behaviour"

Personal issues involved:	Holding back:
• Silence about how senior nurses treat you • "Stay out of trouble" (links with	Distancing as a strategy for managing rejection and painful reprimands.
(Personal issues involved: contd) Fear of reprimand / humiliation) • Fear of rejection / or being pre-judged (links with conforming to try to belong to the ward team and helplessness) • Previous experience not respected by some trained staff.	(Holding back: contd)
Co-variance: About emotional energy:	Holding back:
• High stress levels on the wards (links to helplessness) • Fear of making mistakes • Too much work and too little time to care properly • Poor supervision and poor standards of care. • Finite amount of energy, barely enough for self, and the patients, not also for other nurses • Poor expression of emotions in personal journals, or with other nursing staff	As a strategy for managing emotional energy.

These socio-psychological processes show the links of the emerging categories: helplessness, trusting/ non-trusting and personal vulnerability which could be important factors underlying the development of "the professional shield," that is, the professional distancing on the wards, the with-holding of self in the School of Nursing and the avoidance of intimacy, (see Appendix C) which in itself can be a cause of the above variables at different levels of interpersonal engagement.

In an informal discussion of the research finding, (Chapter 3) I put it to one tutor that nurses had an investment in holding the helpless position in relation to those senior to them as it acted as a good role model for patients. It gave them something in common with patients, in effect, `Look I have to do what I am told, and I want you to do what I tell you, that is how it is in hospital'. The tutor agreed. The reasoning behind the statement was my constant reflective question: what is the investment for nurses (as a profession) in maintaining the status quo with respect to unsatisfactory interpersonal relations which seemed to create a sense of disempowerment? This question will be followed up in the next section, and the salient categories which emerged throughout the whole analysis will be drawn together in the final section of this chapter. Whether this is the research question to come out of this grounded theory study will be discussed in Chapter 7.

Power and control

In this section the issues of power and control within the hierarchical relationship will be explored and how this affected the way nurses related to each other on the wards. To this end the division between this section and the last seems artificial with the main difference being the more positive aspects of expert authority which has been addressed already in this chapter.

Power can be defined in different ways depending on its force and direction, for now two definitions from within an interpersonal perspective are offered by way of starting this analysis. According to Adair & Howell, (1989)

> Power is the ability to do what one chooses, the more power one has the more options one has. Those without power are led to believe this is a personal failing, those with it come to consider it a sign of personal success. (op. cit., p.220)

This definition has implicit within it the value put on the concept of power, so that using power for self can be described as self-empowering and not to have it as disempowering, while using power with others can be either facilitative or coercive as when power is understood as the capacity for one individual or group to mould the behaviour of another individual or group according to the definer's wishes. (Evans, 1978) By control is meant the amount of constraint or coercion used by the power source on the target group as part of the institutionalisation process (to impose conformity to cultural norms) (after Berger and Luckman, 1971, pp.70-89).

One of the first interviewees saw nurses working together in the following light:

> I think there is a lot of cliquishness on the ward. Sometimes it's a group of staff nurses and mature students against the rest of the ward. They can be anti-Sister, or anti-student and sometimes of course they are anti-patient. They can show a front to patients that they all get on well, but when you really work with them and get to know them, there is quite a lot of conflict. (Tutor)

According to Deutsch (1973, p.10) a 'conflict exists whenever incompatible activities occur'. When the conflict is a result of incompatible actions between two or

213

more persons it is called interpersonal or as in the example above intergroup conflict. The above verbatim account is another example of the 'them and us' situation which goes back to the 'belonging' or not belonging to the in-group on the ward. One of the incompatibilities shown in the statement above is managing the "tranquil front" to patients with currents of conflicts bubbling under the surface. This seems like one individual or group- the senior trained staff nurses control the behaviour of others.

During the interviews, there were so many verbatim accounts exposing different facets of the interplay between hierarchy, power and control that it was difficult to differentiate between them. Figure 6.8 is an attempt to show the conceptual links between the three main concepts. The purpose of the illustration is to use verbatim accounts to suggest how their interplay can create conflict in working interpersonal relationships.

Figure 6.8 The relationship between power, control and conflict

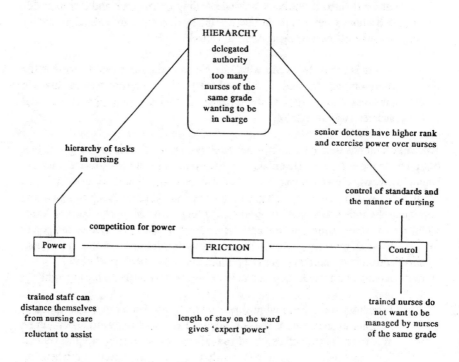

How this conflict manifested itself in the working relation will emerge in the following account, which reflects hierarchical power and control from different perspectives. During one of my observations on a medical ward I asked a student how long she had worked on this general medical ward. She responded:

> I've be working on this ward for 14 weeks now. It's too long... nothing new to learn..things being routine, this is my first experience on acute medicine, although it's my second year of training. People expected me to know more when I came, because I'm a second year. (Student)

This student had worked on her own all morning, however by 11am, all her work was done. She commented:

> I would have liked to have worked with someone else, to be supervised, to have a role model. There is a tension with being a second year student and still have so little experience. When I work on my own and I need help, I have to ask someone to help me, and I'm made to feel inadequate. It feels like you are asking someone to do your work for you.

This relates to the absence of teamwork spoken about previously in this chapter. However, in this section one can interpret the same unsupportive attitude as emerging from inappropriate hierarchical control. The need for a student to have to call out for help and her request for help to be seen as a sign of inadequacy on her part can undermine the student's confidence. The assumption that because she is a second year student she should know about medical nursing and be able to work on her own, shows a lack of sensitivity to her learning needs. There were many such examples of poor use of authority, one being the with-holding of information:

> Likewise, when the Sister does a doctor's round, she will immediately write down any changes on the Care Plan but she won't tell you, you have to find out for yourself. She does not give an overview of general information needed. She is selective about what she tells to whom. They have social meetings, Sister, doctors and social and occupational workers, and you don't know what has been decided. Sometimes you have to ask the patient what is happening to them, you feel a bit of an idiot, not knowing. Patients expect you to know what is to happen to them and you don't always know. (Staff Nurse)

The same state of affairs regarding with-holding of information was recounted by a junior staff nurse on the same ward. Another area of potential conflict for students and trained staff refers to the dilemma of seniority and personal distance versus peer relationships:

There needs to be a gap between staff and students, in how they relate to each other. There should be a distance, a respect, and being here for 16 weeks makes it difficult to keep that distance. The boundaries get blurred, and maybe you get too familiar. Or the staff think so, some staff will speak to me but others don't. Some will say `you must know your place', which can be difficult when we are in small numbers. But it is difficult, to be friendly as well, especially when you work with senior ward staff. They just give orders, but don't do any of the work. I feel used, a pair of hands. Others might feel the same. Staying on the ward too long means that you know the routine, and you relax and maybe don't learn so much. The advantages of staying on the ward for such a long time is that you can communicate more effectively, get familiar with ward routine, and get to know the patients better. The disadvantages are, you get bored with the routine, too familiar with staff, you need to be reminded of your learner status.

This student seems caught in an intrapsychic conflict regarding how she best learns, as well as an interpersonal dilemma about how best to relate to staff. The double messages about personal distance, being friendly, and `being ordered about' can be difficult to juggle. As the student said herself, the boundaries get blurred. This can be a way for those with power to keep those they have power over, in a subservient or uncertain posture which can create anxiety, particularly about `getting it wrong'

Issues of hierarchical control which can cause conflict are many: from being labelled as a problem student before the student even gets on the ward; to fear of reprisal, for example a poor report, as the senior staff are responsible for their references. The phenomenon of your reputation going before you by ward sisters `gossiping' to each other was highlighted by a number of students. One student expressed this fear when she said that one Ward Sister can say to another: `Oh, she is no good...' about learners, before they even come on their wards. This is pre-judging a student from other peoples accounts rather than waiting for experiential evidence for more accurate evaluation. As one Tutor put it:

The poor student is labelled before she even comes on the ward. This causes a lot of stress, making it difficult for students to feel safe and relaxed going onto a new ward if they know such gossip goes on.

Another student graphically illustrated the problems in relationships on the ward:

On the whole I got on well with staff, on the wards, the last ward was my first bad ward. Up till then, I felt that I got on very well with the staff. I was a good team member. All the ward reports showed that they appreciated that, but the last one was very different. As I was near the end

216

of my second year, I felt I knew more about what I am doing, and what is acceptable and what is not acceptable on the ward. This particular ward was very slapdash..

The student nurse then gave a long account of poor nursing, which she was trying not to imitate. She went on to say:

> The staff nurse said `Sister will kill you if she sees you doing that," when the student nurse was trying to do good care. "A lot of things there just were not right. And I found that I was a lot more assertive and I said that I would not accept a poor drug procedure and unfortunately, my standing my ground actually got me a lot of hassle. And the staff were quite unpleasant. A few of them were unpleasant, and a few of them were very friendly to my face, and a lot of bitching behind. And unfortunately, when I got my report, it had some nice things, like I was excellent at my work, but that my choice of priorities was to be looked at. By which they meant that because I did not make the beds before caring for the patients and such like, they didn't like it. The report is all totally contradictory.

The above example shows the inter-relationship between many of the concepts discussed in this chapter, the need to belong to the ward team, the need to conform to be accepted, or at least not to be punished by other nurses and in particular not to have such reprisals as a poor report which will stay on record and be used by the School of Nursing (1) for references purposes. For another student the issue of an unfair ward report because she would not conform to poor practice was not given enough importance by her tutor:

> ...but I mean, in my case when I felt I hadn't got a justified report, one tutor said to me, "Oh, don't worry about it, you've got very good reports all the way, it will just be the same". What the tutor didn't really take into account was how I was actually feeling about it, my self-esteem.

This tutor's response could be taken as an example of learned helplessness, that is, the insolvability of problems regardless of the importance of that problem for the individual.

A rigid hierarchy is maintained throughout the professional strata: from senior doctors to junior doctors, and senior nurses to junior nurses and has been a part of nursing since the Crimean War (Brown 1993). In Smith's (1992) research, when a third year student nurse observed that for the first time there was a more junior nurse on the ward than herself, her comment was `Your not quite the bottom of the dirt pile any more'. (Smith, 1992, p.120) Such a statement indicates that being junior is a distinctive disadvantage to the point of being exploitative. The need to have the respect which goes together with perceived expert authority (position

217

power) is a goal that nurses try to achieve. Remembering from Figure 6.8 that expert authority is assumed or taken by virtue of length of service or the perceived higher status of one group over another rather than real expert knowledge, so needs to be treated with caution.

From a tutor:

> Nurses relate in a subservient way with senior doctors. They usually try to wield power over junior doctors in their own age group. An example is of the junior doctor needing to ask permission from the staff nurse, to read his patient's notes.

According to one tutor:

> Nurses are hierarchically driven. They are afraid of their own breed, because they are trying to get up there with them. They also try to maintain the power with doctors that they have with patients.

This reminds me of patterns of behaviour in oppressed groups, who while being oppressed, say they cannot understand why those in power should treat them in such a manner, yet think that the only way out is to move up from the oppressed position to one of authority themselves and then inflict the same experiences on those junior to, or dependent on them. Such patterns can be found in abusive families, in inter-racial conflict and other institutional and organisational cultures governed autocratically. Some verbatim accounts are offered to identify the conflict or potential conflict between delegated authority and different grades of nursing staff:

> If you have two or three staff nurses on duty together, all wanting to be in charge, in the end, none of them do any work in the ward, which is detrimental to the patients' wellbeing, because they are left with untrained students actually looking after them. (Tutor)

And almost identically from another tutor:

> When you have got three or four staff nurses on the ward they are nearly always in conflict because they are all vying for the power that the senior has and if they are all on duty at the same time, who is the boss? They all wind up in the office shuffling papers while the two students run the ward outside. So increasing the number of qualified staff on the ward has its disadvantages as well. There are too many chiefs and no Indians, so there is a power struggle.

She goes on to say:

I think that nurses think that when they qualify, that is the end of nursing. 'I want to be a manager now.. and I don't want to deal with sick people. I just want to tell people what to do'. There is that element of power, and they become too powerful to deal with patients.

By 'too powerful to deal with patients', this tutor meant that nurses felt too superior to do the ordinary 'basic nursing care' once they qualified. There seemed to be competition to move away from direct patient contact to more prestigious management tasks. This need to move away from direct patient contact confirms that there is a hierarchy of nursing tasks which spans (at the lower end) basic nursing care, to highly technical patient care up to the management of the people doing the nursing care. A theoretical memo in the early stages of the research recorded the issue of power and control, seeing it linked with promotion away from the bedside: away from the physical hard work, less emotional involvement, to having more status, where people will respect them and listen to them. This observation grew stronger with both the ward observations and nurses personal accounts.

What is the power nurses want? Is it to re-gain some measure of self-determinism or to have power-over others which may be a reaction to helplessness or a proactive strategy against helplessness, that is, the need to be part of the decision-making process? The new grading system was instigated to reduce the anomaly of too many senior nurses leaving the clinical areas of nursing for teaching and management positions, however through various political manoeuvres, the grading system turned in on itself to control nurses even more within a hierarchy of grades. The top grades were then 'lost' in political and financial reshuffling, but the grades within the wards stayed. The grading system created more conflict among trained staff by setting up competition between them for promotion through grades without a corresponding change in type of work, for the financial rewards as much as for status. Nurses continued to be allocated tasks according to seniority, rather than by team work or primary nursing in this research hospital. One tutor had a particular slant to her interpretation of non-legitimate authority (abusive power) (Schein, 1988):

I should not be sexist, but I think we see a need for power among women more than men. It may be that men are traditionally more physically powerful and don't need to prove much. I do feel that women strive for power, not all, and these meek little housewives turn into something else in the wards. I think there is a lot of power craziness about.

She went on to say:

It may be something to do with human nature, needing power. Perhaps the powerless woman, the normally powerless woman, enjoying that power. I have often seen this in women...I don't find this with male nurses.

219

It is interesting to try to make sense of the above statements. In Clay (1987) he records that 90 per cent of all entrants are women, yet males dominate the top positions both in nursing and medicine. This tutor seems to believe that women exercising power is a distortion of their role and such behaviour goes against her notions that women should be mild and compliant. This same tutor was the one who felt that she could not confront trained staff about poor standards of care. Clay (1987, p.111) wonders if nurses, particularly women, shy away from seeking 'legitimate power' as it may be linked with 'feminism' as well as with manipulation, abuse or exploitation.

One can see this struggle for power even among senior student nurses and new junior trained staff. For example:

> Students might think, 'I've been on this ward longer than the new staff nurse, I know more about the ward and could challenge the new staff for authority. (Andy)

The notion of 'legitimate authority' and conflict among staff was a feature of one student's concerns. For this student the ward manager and the senior doctors are the right people to confront difficult patients and to manage staff conflict:

> Sister is the captain of the ship. She is there to make sure things run smoothly, to reduce conflict among staff. They should not air their grievance on the ward.

> Sister is best at resolving conflict because she has the authority. It's part of her line management. She should be able to do it. And demanding patients should only be confronted by the Sister or the doctor or staff nurse. Students should complain to trained staff if patients are unreasonable. They can put the patient in his place. (Andy)

The above statement fits with Menzies' (1960, p.19) term 'The reduction of the impact of responsibility by delegation to superiors' as a social defence strategy. Where Menzies was speaking of the devolving of clinical and managerial tasks up the hierarchy, the above student believed that interpersonal relationships which become problematic should also be devolved upwards. To a degree this would be considered appropriate deference to expert authority, but which kind of authority, expert clinical authority or interpersonal relationship skills authority? This research shows that there is a lack of assertion among trained staff as there is among students. If conflict resolution is seen to be the duty of the ward manager, then other nurses do not learn or practise the skills of assertive management, in fact the question begs, how does the ward Sister learn interpersonal assertive management. My experience of teaching Senior Nurses including ward management skills highlighted many areas of weakness in their interpersonal relationship skills, which were detrimental to them as well as to others. The delicate balance of trying to negotiate change among trained staff was highlighted by a staff nurse:

> There are a lot of Grade E's, *(junior trained nurses)* so people are of equal position. So it is best to make suggestions in the form of questions rather than say `I want...' I prefer to say, `Do you think it would be a good idea to...?' This is less dogmatic.

And the wish to manage with so many trained staff on the ward?

> I do a lot of late shifts, so I get a lot of management experience, so I feel ok. Some of the other Grade E's are part time and work mostly on the morning shift. They are a stable group, but as I said the longest one on the ward gets to be in charge, ..but I can be in charge in the evenings.

The hypothesis to be drawn from the above accounts is that power is a form of dependency. Nurses perceive patients to be psychologically and often physically depending on them (for ward routines, control of information and regimentation) and they in their turn are depended on others in authority. This is likened to Menzies' (1960, pp.16-17) category "Collusive social redistribution of responsibility and irresponsibility." According to Menzies nurses find the responsibility of their role so intrapsychically stressful, that they project it outward mainly as an interpersonal conflict about each other's ability to take `proper' responsibility, that is hierarchical authority and power. The findings in this study supports Menzies' assertion that nurses' need to keep the rigid hierarchical structures in place, and maintain a certain amount of interpersonal conflict as a way of managing intrapersonal stress. This pattern of behaviour also knits well with the hypothesis I shared with a tutor of nurses role-modelling to patients how to be dependent. As Sines (1993) said, "Managers dominate the front-line workers who, in turn, dominate their clients". Yet the written philosophical statement in nursing care in the research hospital was the intention of `sharing power with patients and their relatives'. The concept of primary nursing was to build up a working contract between a patient and his /her nurse in which both are in partnership in the management of illness to health for the patients. My contention is that for more equal power sharing between nurse and patient the whole working ambience needs to encourage nurses to work co-operatively with each other as well as with patients and that this needs to be demonstrated experientially among nurses themselves. Given all the constraints mentioned in this chapter so far, nurses would need a high degree of political and social awareness to do this as well as being able and willing to function at a skilled interpersonal level with peers, seniors and patients. It is here where the link to the educational intentions for nurses to be personally and interpersonally competent meets the interpersonal demands of their work. And yet, what was often found in this study can be summed up in one tutor's comment:

> Nurses are... hierarchically controlled, historically, a servant girl ethos. Religious ethos., both were devoted and subservient.

That was a tutor's statements about nurses. Do tutors inadvertently pass on this historical attitude about how to be a nurse to their students? Nurses say that they have very little influence on the wards, and blame organisational changes or the hierarchical nature of the working structure. The psychodynamic environment on the ward is considered to be the relationship between nurses working in a way that fosters a meaningful and enhancing relationship for all concerned and which allows the development of the personality to maturity. It addresses the issues of conflict and interpersonal problems, using creative strategies to effect solutions.
But, as one student put it,

> It is up to the Sister or the Charge Nurse on the ward to say: `I am in position of responsibility, and I must have a happy team and changes will need to be made.

> JG: So changes to the interpersonal dynamic can be initiated and sustained within the ward nursing team?

> Student: Well, I think it can, I have always had great evidence of that in psychiatry.

> JG: You have had evidence of that in terms of, you were able to get the team to be working happily together, that was different from how the structure was, not different, but that you could separate them out?

> Student: Absolutely, yes. Sister was in control. Now when I say control I don't mean it to sound that Sister was an autocrat, because she was not, she was a very democratic individual, but if things weren't going right on the ward then a ward meeting would be called. You see, we always had very regular ward meetings where people were encouraged to say what they were not happy about and get it thrashed out at work. If the line manager then had to become involved, if things arose which had to go to a higher level, well then it did. But the Ward Sister or Charge Nurse has got a tremendous responsibility.

> JG: It seems from what you are saying that, in terms of team, or group dynamics on the ward, it is possible to make substantial changes about how people are with each other at that level?

Student: Yes, it is.

The important focus of the above questioning was to ascertain whether the nurse felt that the ward team had any power to influence change at a local level rather than expect change at an interpersonal level to come from outside the wards. I also wanted to check through theoretical sampling whether the fear of reprimand kept the nurses in a state of conformity, or whether it was lack of assertion skills, or both. I asked the above student:

> JG: People see poor standards and say they are frightened to challenge trained staff for fear of retaliation. Is that an imagined fear or real when students say well they (the trained staff) have got to write my cards and the end or my report, is that a realistic fear?

> Student: I think in some cases, yes, I think it depends on the individual member of trained staff. Some will do things in a certain way because they have always done them that way. For example, let's say you saw a trained nurse sitting a patient on a ring to relieve pressure areas. Let's say a student approached her and said, "In line with recent research, this should not be practised now," and she was able to back that up, and suggest another way of doing it which is more in keeping with how things are done now. Now then, some trained staff would be able to accept that and listen, but some wouldn't. It is these people who are very set in their ways and lack communication skills themselves, maybe resentful of advice coming from a student.

> JG: Is it realistic that the retaliation could happen?

> Student: Oh, yes.. oh, yes. definitely. I personally have seen it happen. It has never happened to me, it has been tried with me. I have always used a professional approach and said, you must give me specific incidents.

> JG: So you have actually problem solved the situation..

> Student: Oh, yes, and they can't do it.

> JG: They can't go into the problem solving and say "well it happened...?

> Student: No they can't...

> JG: So that seems to be all part of your assertion skills, some one starts accusing you, you actually say `ok..when did this happen?

223

Student: Specific incidence, and why didn't you tell me immediately. It all boils down to, they will try to get you back, because they don't like your attitude, or they don't like the fact that you challenged them in some way, or brought something to their attention that they haven't appreciated... (Student)

This student had learned assertion skills as a psychiatric nurse before the general nurse training she was doing during the time of this interview. I reflected with her that the more I thought about what underlies assertion in terms of personal confidences and self image, the more I saw this as a difficulty for junior nurses if the ward environment was punitive, and leading to undermining self-confidence. The student agreed.

The following account specifically looks at the friction caused between senior staff nurses and a junior staff nurse. It is a particularly painful account, and gives an indication of the lengths people will go to when wanting to control others. During ward observations (Chapter 3) (Gregory 1994), this ward seemed the most stable, not too easy going nor too rigid in its management style. On the surface there seemed little to disturb the stability of the ward, yet I had heard from a tutor that students did have a difficult time on this ward. Why they might do so can be deduced from the account which follows: Kate, a staff nurse:

The senior staff won't tell you what is going on, they intimidate you, and it is just absolutely impossible. Well I mean I have met some people who are impossible, but I have never come across any one like that before, *(laughs)* and there is just nothing you can do. I mean, I went to her when I had been here two and a half weeks and I had everything knocked right out of me, all my stuffing knocked right out of me, my cheerfulness, my ideas of things, everything just knocked dead... and I just couldn't stand it any more, being abused in front of people, in front of patients and doctors, being shouted at and one thing and another.. just feeling like... Why am I here, there is no reason for me to be here, not doing anything valuable. I may as well be an auxiliary and the NHS would save a couple of thousand pounds a year. So I thought I would be really diplomatic about it and I would take her aside, somewhere quiet where no one can hear and I would just say, in quiet tones and everything, that she makes me unhappy and that I don't want to work with her any more, unless things change, which I did, and she just hit the roof, she went absolutely mad, screaming and shouting and all of it was a load of rubbish, like she mumbles all the words together so you can't hear what she is saying anyway. Obviously she didn't know what to say so she was screaming and shouting and I was really upset. I was crying and the patients noticed, and I went on to the balcony and stayed out there for a bit.

224

I felt that I didn't know where to turn at all, I didn't know .. like when you are a student, you know you have always got the school, you know that you can always go there, you can always walk off the ward and go there, because you are not accountable- for your actions when you are a student. Well I couldn't go walking off the ward, so I thought I will ring the Nursing Officer and talk to her. I went to ring her, and who should be talking to the Nursing Officer but this other nurse *(laughs)* she beat me to it. The next day I spoke to Sister about it. I had a long chat with her, we had this other nurse in the room as well, and she sat there and lied, she was absolutely lying about dates and incidents that had occurred, patient's names, and she lied, saying she had done something she had not done. And I was going "your lying, your lying" (laughs). and I just cried my eyes out, and I thought, I've got to get out.

Since then it has not been quite so bad, because this person almost completely ignores me. Occasionally, when she is forced to speak to me, she is reasonably polite. But it is the atmosphere here more than anything.

JG: It feels like it took a lot of courage for you to do that, to call this person aside, and then to say how you were feeling about things.

Kate: I am not afraid of anybody. I didn't think twice about doing that, I would do that with anybody, but I have never had to do that before. I had one incident when I had problems with her, and I could not do any more to help her. This staff nurse was dangerous, they usually are, they are usually incompetent and dangerous and they need to make things bad for everyone else, maybe it is their own inadequacy, I don't know what it is.

JG: What do you mean by dangerous?

Kate: Dangerous can mean when they don't want to learn any more, and they don't know anything anyway, therefore they have got no knowledge to be on a ward and they don't want to learn either.

JG: You were saying, that you wanted to ring the Nursing Officer and get some support, and she was already communicating with the other nurse, and subsequently, were you able to find any support?

Kate: From junior members of staff, students I mean. Like I am a junior member of the staff, as in qualified. There was one lady that used to visit the ward from the School, and I used to have a good old moan to her. She comes up occasionally, she is really nice. And I bought a book, called 'The Staff Nurse Survival Guide'.

225

JG: Oh, really, Oh, right. I haven't seen that. So you didn't find a lot of help from the senior managers, or were you not able to ask for it?

Kate: Only the Sister, and she was very nice at the time in the office, but as soon as you left the office, it was nothing else. There was no further support, at least I didn't think there was.

JG: How long has the senior staff team been on this ward?

Kate: I am not sure. I think it has been quite a while, I think about eleven years or so.

JG: Eleven years? That's quite a long time. If you have got a caring environment like when you felt you were valued, as you have just mentioned, what effect does it have, if any, on how you are with patients?

Kate: No, I think it makes it better. Because the way it is now, when I am on with that Staff Nurse I am having problems with, it is like there is a huge gap between us, and it is obvious to see, anybody can see it. I am sure that the patients have noticed today, they are bound to have. I can't explain it. It is difficult to explain, I think there is a much nicer atmosphere when myself and one of the other girls are on together.

JG: Are the patients actually cared for better?

Kate: I would say so, yes, in terms of quality and quality of care. Definitely, quality, because myself and the other two nurses work together, even if one of them is in charge. Because if I am on with either of them, because they are more senior, they are in charge, as there are only two trained permanent nurses on per shift, but they don't just sit at the desk doing paper work, they will come and give me a hand. Isn't it better for patients to be nursed by trained staff who are happy working together than by untrained staff?

Such obvious interpersonal conflict as expressed by Kate is difficult to countenance in a profession which calls itself caring. Many of the controlling variables which operated between student and trained staff, such as assessment of performance and ward reports with the fear of reprisal around these would not feature in the relationship between these staff nurses and yet because of the seniority between them the incidents of mis-use of positional power (Schein, 1988) is not resolved.

From whichever perspective the ward conflict has been studied in this research the underlying basic sociopsychological process of managing personal vulnerability seem to be at work. Psychosocial elements such as insecurity amongst colleagues regarding what is culturally rewarded within the (ward) organisation; the bias towards clinical knowledge over interpersonal relationship management; the power given to hierarchical status; common goals and methods of working together show a level of personal vulnerability which the nurses try to protect against. This level of vulnerability confirms for those in the experience their need to be self-protective which they manifest through 'Professional shield' behaviour. In the final section of this chapter the intention is to bring all the salient categories together to identify the core categories and the basic sociopsychological processes with which nurses have been engaged in interpersonally.

Core categories and basic socio-psychological processes

In this section the main salient categories making up the core categories and the sociopsychological processes will be illustrated. The intention is to integrate the categories which offer an emerging theory of interpersonal relationships among nurses in the general hospital setting and how nurse education influences these relationships.

From Chapter 4 it can be seen that the core category identified was 'With-holding self as a strategy for self-management'. The tension is between 'Belonging in the learning set' with the necessary sub-categories; peer group support, trusting self, disclosing self and mutual feedback forming the pillars of 'Belonging in the learning set' in their positive dimensions and with-holding self when the criteria for feeling psychologically safe were not met. Figure 4.6 showed what elements needed to be in place to create a positive group learning environment, and Figure 4.7 illustrate the elements found in the negative group learning environment which fostered the strategy of 'With-holding self as a strategy for self-management'.

On the following page the various categories can be put together in an attempt to map the sociopsychological picture of how nurses manage their vulnerability in the face of difficult complex educational and working based relationships.

Figure 6.9 **Mapping the elements of the substantive theory of 'With-holding self as a strategy for self management'**

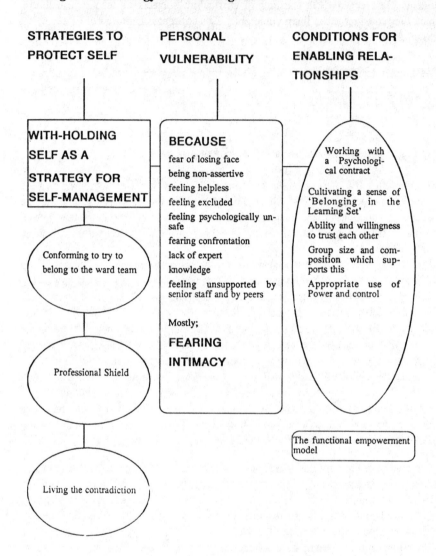

STRATEGIES TO
PROTECT SELF

PERSONAL
VULNERABILITY

CONDITIONS FOR
ENABLING RELA-
TIONSHIPS

WITH-HOLDING
SELF AS A
STRATEGY FOR
SELF-MANAGEMENT

BECAUSE
fear of losing face
being non-assertive
feeling helpless
feeling excluded
feeling psychologically unsafe
fearing confrontation
lack of expert
knowledge
feeling unsupported by
senior staff and by peers

Mostly;
FEARING
INTIMACY

Working with
a Psychologi-
cal contract

Cultivating a sense of
'Belonging in the
Learning Set'

Ability and willingness
to trust each other

Group size and com-
position which sup-
ports this

Appropriate use of
Power and control

Conforming to try to
belong to the ward team

Professional Shield

Living the contradiction

The functional empowerment
model

This with-holding of self is more than emotional distancing or detachment (Marshall, 1980) as it embraces cognitive and behavioural attributes as well. Students close down their learning in curriculum subjects or teaching methods which they consider make them vulnerable. This concept is captured in Figure 6.10 below:

Figure 6.10 The negative feedback loop (after Paton, et. al., 1985)

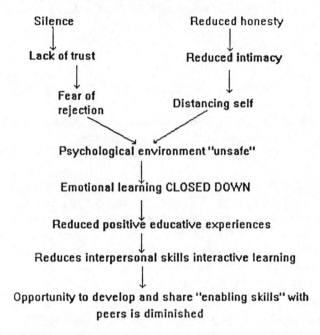

The consequence of such a close-down is that learners are trained as technologists rather than " Enablers" (therapeutic agents).

The School of Nursing had placed itself and its staff in the unenviable position of 'Living the contradiction' of the two educations; education from above and the education of equals.(Chapter 4) The tutors' (apart from one) strategy for managing this contradiction was also to distance themselves, particularly from educational interactive experiential teaching methods.

In Chapter 6 the main core categories with auxiliary categories have been 'Conforming to try to belong to the ward team' with its many sub-categories illustrated in Figure 6.1. The category; 'Professional shield' with its sub-categories was significant as a strategic basic socio-psychological process. These socio-psychological processes, derived from a sense of personal vulnerability encountered both in the educational environment which was seen to be psychologically 'unsafe' and the ward because of the conflict around power and control when synthesised, offer the following core processes:

- The `Professional shield' (see Figure 6.7) with the with-holding of trust by individuals in what was perceived to be an un-supportive working environment.

Some of the many ways in which nurses felt vulnerable are listed below, taken from theoretical memos:

Personal vulnerability:

- coping on their own on the wards-difficulty in asking for support from peers and seniors
- fear of humiliation, both on the wards if reprimanded in public and in the School of Nursing if they express their emotions
- distancing themselves from traumatic events, covering up own fear?

Personal vulnerability per se would not automatically lead to `With-holding as a strategy for self management', as emotionally competent people would both manage the vulnerability and engage in encounters with others for the purposes of personal learning and achievement of intended outcomes. However, personal vulnerability compounded by elements of helplessness and a punitive hierarchy create such a level of intrapsychic stress that the person may well demonstrate with-holding behaviour. Ultimately this leads to the principle core process of:

Fearing intimacy in the form of openness about self and honesty with others.

This is the core category which is not so much a socio-psychological process but rather a state of being which is the result of poor educative experiences, personal disrespect and lack of interpersonal support. To manage this state of being nurses engage in the basic socio-psychological process:

With-holding of self as a strategy for self-management

The concept of intimacy here is the one derived from the theory of Transactional Analysis. Amongst other things, this personality and communications theory offers a framework about how people structure time. Of the seven ways that Berne (1964, p.160) defined how people structure their time, intimacy is the one which is distress-free, which is psychologically healthy as the people involved are not using time and interpersonal relationships to act out, either by avoidance, or reaction, some previously distressing situation. (This links with Heron's (1992) definition of

230

emotional competence. (Chapter 1) Intimacy is about expressing authentic feelings and wants without censoring. In intimacy, there are no secret messages. The social level and the psychological level are congruent. In intimacy, you make it as clear as you can what you want through emotions as well as words, on a feeling as well as a thinking level. The effectiveness of the communication can be 100%.

The word intimacy as used by Berne is specialised to do with communication and is different from intimacy in a physical or sexual sense. Psychological games which are distressed forms of communicating needs and wants are a substitute for intimacy; a way of getting human recognition by exploitation without taking personal responsibility for the outcome. Intimacy is the most risky of all ways of time structuring as we are communicating without discounting each other, therefore the outcome of intimacy should always be constructive for the people concerned. However they may not always find it comfortable, as this depends on the mix or not of honest affirmations (positive strokes) or constructive criticism (negative strokes) [10](Berne 1972) and their intensity.

However intimacy is only one of the qualities of the autonomous individual. The others are self-awareness and spontaneity (Berne 1964). All three are interrelated, hence the need for self-awareness as a pre-requisite to developing any distress-free enabling relationship. As intimacy involves personal risk, therefore triggering personal vulnerability, it will usually only emerge in psychologically safe interpersonal relationships. The risk is to the self esteem. In Chapters 4 and 5 much of the 'holding back' in experiential learning and interpersonal skills was through fear of losing face. Much of the 'holding back' in the wards is for the same reason, that is, being reprimanded in public and excluded from the ward team. The greater the perceived risk, (to self-esteem) the greater the holding back. The less the perceived risk (of attack to self-esteem) the more open involvement people will engage in, both in learning and in working on the ward.

Being empathically supportive of another person implies a level of intimacy, which the nurses I interviewed said they were not encouraged to have with peers. They were also unsure what intimacy meant and whether they wanted that kind of relationship with colleagues. Intimacy is about supporting each other in vulnerability, yet none want to be seen to be vulnerable.

Conclusion

In this chapter the focus has been the interpersonal dynamic between nurses working on general wards. The ward observations told a story of busy nurses who worked along side each other in what seemed a collaborative way. However it proved so difficult to 'get behind' the work front to tap into the nurses interpersonal relationships that this form of data collecting was put to one side in preference for indepth interviews and informal discussions. The disappearing nurses during slack times, particularly over lunch lends support to the emerging theory of 'With-holding of self as a strategy for self-management', the management of their fear of intimacy in the face of a culture which did not seem to know what intimacy meant, how it should be manifested behaviourally and perhaps to a lesser degree, in beliefs, values, thinking and emotions.

This chapter looked at some of the issues causing a fear of intimacy of which Figure 6.9 is a summary. These included the need to conform, the fear of reprisals, the power struggles which caused interpersonal conflict and the personal vulnerability creating a professional shield as the main strategy for with-holding self in interpersonal relationships.

Notes

8   Teamwork: Establishment of interdependence of tasks and skills with people supporting the achievement of goals through group actions.

9   Enrolled nurses trained for two years to be assistant nurses to the Registered Nurse.

10   Strokes are defined by Berne (1972, p.23) as units of recognition which means that all verbal and non-verbal recognition interactions have a value, perceived to be either positive or negative, for the people involved.

7   Conclusion

Introduction

This chapter concludes the research exploring the interpersonal relationships amongst nurses both in the School of Nursing and in the General Hospital wards of one district hospital. The question of how education for interpersonal relating influences the way nurses relate to each other both in the School of Nursing and on the wards has been answered in many ways, even if obliquely. In essence, by virtue of not explicitly educating for interpersonal relating, whether social or therapeutic, the School mirrored the ambivalence which prevailed about interpersonal relating both in the School and on the wards.

Many possible reasons were found for this in this research and a summary of the integrated findings will be given before going on to evaluate the research and make recommendations for implementation of the findings. Suggestions for further research will also be offered.

Summary of the research

In Chapter 1, the groundwork was laid for exploring the subject of interpersonal relationships within the conceptual frame of humanistic principles and practice. (Rowan 1988) Nurse education, as part of moving away from a skills based apprentice training syllabus (GNC 1977) aligned itself gradually during the 1980s with an educational philosophy which could also find application and relevance in nursing practice, that is, a humanistic philosophy (Peplau 1988, Townsend 1983a, Marson 1985, Beverley 1988). This philosophy, under the banner of "empowerment", paralleled the move towards an individualistic and consumer driven ideology within the wider social and political arena which expanded the concept of empowerment of individuals to distinctive groups. This person-centred approach has culminated in the last decade in such political projects as the Conventions on the Rights of the Child (Children's rights) adopted by the United

Nations General Assembly (1989), and nationally by the "Working for Patients" (HMSO 1989), the Parent's Charter (Dept. of Education 1991, 1994), and so on, under the broad umbrella of the Citizen's Charter formulated in the United Kingdom in 1991 (HMSO 1991). Nurse education was in the forefront of professional education, introducing such a philosophy into the public arena through its endorsement of humanistic beliefs, values and practices in the Registered Mental Nurse Syllabus of 1982. (GNC 1982). Within this person-centred approach to education and to nursing, the social and psychological aspects of learning and caring began to take equal place with behaviour (skills) based training and task-focused clinical nursing within curriculum documents under the broad perspective of holism. (Pearson & Vaughan, 1986, Beattie, 1987, Bevis, 1989)

Within the nursing curriculum, social and psychological theories were most appropriately introduced within the social and psychological aspects of care and the interpersonal relations dimension which nurses needed to engage in as part of the patient-centred nursing care models. (King, 1971, RCN, 1987, Peplau, 1988, Orem, 1980). This had particular urgency as the research literature of the 1970s and 1980s strongly advocated for nurses to have `better' communication skills; to give more time to meeting patients psychosocial needs and for trained nurses to develop more facilitative skills when educating both junior nurses (student nurses particularly) and their patients (Ashworth, 1980, Kagan, et. al., 1986 and others) (see Chapter 1). This consensus within the profession that the interpersonal relationship between the nurse and patient was central to the definition of nursing was seen as a unifying process which carried with it the optimism of humanism itself.

During the 1980s many nurse educationalists and practitioners could see the merging of humanistic values and practices within nurse education and nursing practice within the UK, which were reflected in the sociocultural need of consumers, that is, patients. However, in retrospect, one can see that such a blending of values and practices to create a caring therapeutic environment was sporadic, relying more on individual vision or highly specialised nursing areas where people were recruited and trained in such values and practices. Such places included some modern acute psychiatric units, some Hospices, some midwifery units, some acute intensive care units and AID's care units, in fact the humanistic educational `movement' was effected through post-registration training. What still needed to be done was to bring such teaching and nursing practice into the pre-registration educational programme for all student nurses. This is where this research has its origins (Chapter 1) and the research progressed on the premise that if nursing is accepted as a psychosocial therapeutic process and given equal importance as clinical caring, then the study of nurses' perceptions and practices of psychosocial therapeutic aspects of nursing is a significant area of study for all nurses and particularly those who would educate students for this aspect of their work.

To remain consistent with the humanistic approach espoused in nurse education the definition of the educated person offered by Heron (1974) (Chapter 1) and supported by Jarvis (1986) was used as a template on which to compare the

234

education of nurses. This definition was used as it both matched the definition of the education of adults and the qualities sought in a professional therapeutic agent (Rogers, 1983) as espoused in the S.O.N. curriculum documents (1986, 1990). Such personal agency was also made explicit by the UKCC (1986) as it exhorted nurses to be responsible autonomous practitioners being morally and organisationally responsible for their practice. Measured against this definition nurses, in this study, were found not to be educated people with respect to their interpersonal relationships at work. Many nurses did not have a sense of personal agency (Harré 1983), that is: they did not feel they were in possession of an ultimate power of decision and action, they did not feel self-directing in negotiating the curriculum content to address their interpersonal relationship needs, or know how to use the educational opportunities to facilitate their learning in psychosocial skills. Equally, many of the students and some of the junior trained staff reported feeling helpless to influence change on the ward, or very stressed conforming to the ward culture. Nurses, both students and junior staff nurses, felt they were at the receiving end of other people's whims and management style (Chapter 6). Nurses in this study felt they had to follow their seniors' beliefs, norms and practices about the place and quality of interpersonal relating within the context of the ward routine and this dimension seemed to create much interpersonal conflict among the nursing staff. They did not feel empowered to set their own criteria for therapeutic relationship behaviour but rather experienced being socialised into each ward's milieu where sanctions operated to encourage conformity to the prevailing cultural norms. It followed then that if nurses were not self-directing then the skills of self-monitoring and self-correction did not operate as an educative process, rather nurses used these reflective skills to monitor their conformity to ward practice through a process of self-stereotyping (Turner, 1987). The nurses' attention and motivation were shifted away from improving their therapeutic relationships towards learning how to `fit in' (Melia, 1987) on every ward they went to.

Revisiting core categories - The basic socio-psychological process

As part of exploring the educational background to this research some issues of concern were identified regarding the attempted merger of the traditional educational approach with the personal-centred andragogical practice (Knowles, 1978, ENB. 1987) more suited to the education of health care professionals. (S.O.N. (1) 1989). Jarvis' (1986) description of the two educations proved to be a robust model with which the relationships within the learning environment in the School of Nursing could be compared and analysed. The nature of the category `Living the contradiction' demonstrated the interface between `old ways of doing things' and the `newer ways' which was found to approximate Jarvis' `education from above and the education of equals'.

235

The School of Nursing where this research took place, moved between the two educations in its curricular documents showing a bias for the `education from above' although it advocated the `education of equals' (Jarvis, 1986). There are others in nurse education who advocate a mixing of what is best in both curricular models (Beattie, 1987), a mixture which Jarvis did not perceive as possible ideologically, but which he recognised as a tension existing in nurse education. This tension was identified by the tutors in this study when they spoke of education of the person at a process level, and education for the profession as a product. (UKCC. Rule 18 competence based training (1983)). In many ways the School of Nursing attempted to emulate Stenhouse's (1975) process curriculum model, with a cocktail mixture of Schon's (1983) concepts of the reflective practitioner, Knowles (1972) and Rogers' (1983) approach to adult education, with a pinch of experiential approaches to learning following Steinaker & Bell (1979). The educational philosophy stated that it wished to focus on the development of attributes and skills in self-direction, assertiveness and confidence in students' interpersonal relating in their nursing role and to their ability to be problem-solvers in clinical matters. (S.O.N.(1) 1986) For this to happen in practice the wards' philosophy and practice towards learners would need to be the same as the School of Nursing's, that is, encouraging reflective self-directed learning with the freedom to explore and experiment necessary to develop independent responsible practitioners (Holden, 1991), and this proved a weak link in the ideological chain. The notion of `fitting in' highlighted by Melia (1987) could not be considered as an empowerment strategy, rather the opposite, at a process level, that is, how nurses managed the dis-empowerment; the very nature of the `fitting in' was the behavioural manifestation of the philosophical conflict between nurse education and nursing practice on the wards. Melia identified the "fitting in" as one of compliance. Such compliance is an indicator of the stress on nurses as a result of the clash of values between the education of the person and education for the professional role. (Dewey, 1938, Jarvis, 1986) (see Chapter 1) A protective passive strategy to such stress would be compliance to the dominant culture with which one wants to identify with. (Turner, et. al., 1987)

In this clash of values, one can understand what is meant by the "espoused theory" and the "theory-in-use". From Paton's interpretation of Argyris' (1964) theory, Paton commented that:

> The espoused theory can differ markedly from the theory-in-use. The significance of this distinction is that most organisations *(including educational organisations)* are run in such a way as to produce a level of psychological immaturity in most of their members. There are not adequate opportunities for individuals to enhance their self-esteem by being psychologically successful and most leaders treat their subordinates in ways which depreciate their creativity, intelligence and abilities. This is the theory-in-use. (Paton, et. al., 1985, p.94)

236

In education, the theory-in-use remained firmly within Tyler's (1949) behavioural and Bruner's (1972) cognitive curriculum models, blending behavioural objectives with propositional knowledge within a medical perspective of clinical (nursing) practice. This ambivalence between the theory-in-use and the espoused theory influenced the importance that both tutors and students gave to the principles of the `education of equals'. Yet, it is under the umbrella of the education of equals where the self-directed person most learns the skills of interpersonal relating. They did this by developing the skills of assessing and articulating personal needs, defining learning objectives to meet those needs, setting personal and group competence based standards and working through a self, peer and tutor assessment (Kilty, 1978). These processes offer opportunities for the learner and tutor to develop many of the skills in interpersonal relating: from self-awareness to assertiveness; emotional competence including stress management; the understanding of different power dimensions; the management of conflict; and the ability to relate to others in a spontaneous and honest fashion. In the absence of such spontaneous relationships the core category identified in educational interactions was: `With-holding of self as a strategy for self-management.

This with-holding of self was seen as a way of managing interpersonal environments which were perceived to be personally vulnerable for those in the situation. In Chapter 4 the many possible factors influencing why students found the educational environment psychologically unsafe, particularly in group learning, were identified and discussed. Equally there was much evidence from small groups of what constituted a psychologically safe supportive learning group as also from one fairly large group of students I observed (16 people) These were important counter-arguments (see Figure 4.6 `The positive group learning environment') , which supported the finding, as the qualities which they identified as conducive to a psychologically safe environment were those missing in the unsafe learning environment (Figure 4.7, `The negative group learning environment'). From this the analysis looked at the need for explicit boundaries around interactive and experiential groupwork to facilitate optimal learning and offered the concept of the psychological contract. The notion of a psychological contract is not new to this study (Paton, et. al., 1985, Minardi & Riley 1988), although the need for one arose out of this research data and the factors which make up the contract were a direct result of the analysis of the data. Kagan (1985) spoke indirectly of the psychological contract in nurse education when she said:

> The tutor-student relationship will have to be founded on non-defensiveness, openness and honesty , and this in turn means that tutors will have to acquire new and often threatening teaching skills. (Kagan, 1985, p.291)

The `new and often threatening skills' Kagan referred to are those which tutors need to facilitate through experiential learning of interpersonal skills in a groupwork environment. (Figure 4.9)

One of the significant findings of the study was the uncertainty among tutors about managing group learning and understanding the group psychosocial dynamic as it unfolded over time. The point to be made here is that most interactive groups go through various stages of forming, storming and norming as they move towards performing as an effective group, which is a healthy process in group development (Tuckman, 1965, Worchel, et. al., 1992). More awareness of normal group development and the necessary skills to facilitate interactive or experiential groups was absent amongst the tutoring staff of the School of Nursing. I believe that the tutors at this School were being ethical in their professional stance, that is, they perceived the moral significance of their educational role, and used their free will to put into action and take responsibility only for that part of the curriculum which they had knowledge and experience of, leaving out either content or methods which they felt they were "not trained for". Most of these tutors felt unable to do full justice to experiential ways of teaching interpersonal skills so they did the minimum to maintain rapport with students and kept to the curriculum contract they felt `safe with'. In this way, tutors also demonstrated a with-holding of self to actively engage in teaching students how best to manage the curriculum to meet their learning needs.

The with-holding of self as a strategy for managing personal vulnerability is like the distancing found in Menzies' (1960) work between nurses and patients. In this research this `with-holding' was found to occur between student nurses themselves and between junior and senior nurses. The issue of trust between nurses was a major factor underlying the need to be self-protective. Nurses' lack of trust for each other surfaced most in experiential groupwork and other participative learning situations, where discussions of interpersonal issues between students, with the giving and receiving of feedback created fears of negative appraisal and even fears of negative motivation behind positive affirmations. It would be easy to say that the lack of trust was due to the students' inexperience in expressing themselves in groupwork, or that nurses perceived groupwork and interpersonal skills training as irrelevant, however, this was not seen to be the case. What was a significant finding was the critical, and for some, punitive environment in which they worked, which then influenced their behaviour. (see Figure 4.7 in Chapter 4) To counter-balance the negative group dynamic in group learning, students spoke of the elements needed for them to feel psychologically safe. Elements under the broad category of `Belonging in the learning set' (Figure 4.9. in Chapter 4) coupled with the psychological contract" between the tutor and students to facilitate individual learning (Figure 4.8 in Chapter 4). This was seen as a way of reducing the perceived need for nurses and tutors to use the strategy of with-holding self as a strategy for self-management, that is, managing their vulnerability.

It became clear in this study that interpersonal relationships among nurses, both in the School of Nursing, and to a greater extent in the wards was the major cause of stress and disillusionment both for student nurses and junior staff nurses. It is difficult for me to say that the interpersonal relationships were poor, rather, although the relationships seemed to be self-regenerating between the people concerned, it was un-educative (in the Deweyan sense (1938)) in many respects. Much of the conflict in interpersonal relationships was seen to be caused by enforced competitive, hierarchical practice and a series of discounting systems (Steiner 1990) which seemed to be in place. Student nurses wanted to be given the same respect as they saw given to trained staff and to patients, and junior staff nurses wanted the same. (Fig. 6.5 in Chapter 6) Those nurses I interviewed felt that their own emotional needs were not being met, so felt unable or unwilling to give emotional support to patients, relatives and other nurses. All agreed that nursing is an interpersonal relationship which `should' be enabling, or have the quality of caring. They felt however that their ability to practise enabling interpersonal relations was dependent on:

1   the ward culture
2   the role modelling they received
3   how enabled they felt themselves to be
4   their skills in interpersonal relationships, particularly their ability to act as agent on behave of self, (in the Harré sense) and their uncertainty about how interpersonal conflict should be managed.

The core category of: `Conforming to try to belong to the ward team' was a salient feature of ward culture. The need to understand the culture of the ward, the prioritising between tasks and nursing process as a caring quality was significant. The argument I put forward is that nursing `as a doing to patients' needs a belief and values base which must have a moral imperative if nursing is to change to `a nursing with patients' and also that the moral imperative of caring needs to extend to those who nurse as well as those who are nursed. This was borne out by research participants' views that the quality of care they gave to patients was influenced by the quality of care they felt they received from peers and senior nurses. To facilitate caring relationships among nurses themselves the Functional Empowerment Model (Roberts, 1993) was offered as an organisational working model, complementary to the psychological contract needed in the educational environment. These two models illustrate the parallel processes influencing nurses' relationships with each other at an intrapsychic level as well as interpersonally. Both models are saying the same thing, that is, that psychological safety is the bedrock on which individuals and groups either flourish or wither. Helplessness (Seligman, 1975, Salvage, 1985) is one consequence of a dysfunctional organisational system, which is both a consequence of the system and feeds it as a negative feedback loop maintaining the status quo. (Paton, et. al., 1985, p.36) Psychological safety in the work place is then a necessary requirement if nurses are to feel confident and comfortable to learn and practise their "enabling skills".

The fact that nurses do not feel psychologically safe despite all the research and education of nurse managers and tutors leads to the hypothesis that there might be an investment in holding on to the status quo. One rationale could be that unconsciously the investment in remaining powerless and psychologically unsafe is that it helps in "winning over patients" that is, to make it easier for patients to trust nurses. The identification issue "we are all weak, or we are both (patients and students) victims together" is a strong one. The belief could be that powerless nurses act as good role models to patients, it gives patients permission to be dependent on nurses as it gives junior nurses permission to be dependent on `higher authority'.Is this cultural? Such `collective (conscious?) powerlessness' links very strongly with Menzies' (1960) category "Collusive social redistribution of responsibility and irresponsibility". Menzies asserted that nurses found taking on the responsibility of their role intrapsychically painful, particularly over a sustained period, and wanted to `abandon their role'. Their way of managing the conflict was to project it out as interpersonal conflict amongst themselves, which was manifested in blaming behaviour. That is, seniors blaming juniors for being irresponsible, and juniors complaining, "that their seniors as a category, impose unnecessary strict and repressive discipline and treat them as though they have no sense of responsibility" (ibid., 1960, p.17). Menzies' words of 34 years ago were echoed in this research and are being stressed here as they directly confront the idea of nurse education addressing the education of the person, as it did not seem so in this study. The educated person works on self to be emotionally competent and not displace the intrapsychic distress onto others whether colleagues or patients. (Heron 1974). Jung's (1977) notion of the "shadow", that is, aspects of self not liked and accepted by the individual creates the intrapsychic conflict and needs to be worked through to a sense of self-acceptance to enable nurses as with other therapeutic agents (Hawkins & Shohet, 1989, p.8) to be as distress-free as is possible when facilitating psychosocial care and change in others.

The opposite end of the bipolar construct of helplessness is power and how it is perceived and used. Paton (1985, p.63) speaks of the overlap between `positional power, expert power, dependency power and personal power'. All shades of power are appropriate in relationships when managed consciously and constructively, and are inappropriate if used coercively (Bennis, et. al., 1976) This relates to the use and abuse of power spoken of in Chapter 6. where the very nature of the hierarchical system can encourage a power-coercive (op cit.) management strategy. Many nursing papers have discussed the power dimension within nursing, (Ashley, 1973, Kratz, 1984, Carlson-Catalano, 1992, Wilmot, 1993, Farmer, 1993 to name a few) most of which touch on the emerging theory of this research, which is that nurses:

> Fear intimacy in the form of openness about self and honesty with others and use `With-holding of self as a strategy for self-management'

The power or perceived lack of power was highlighted by Ashley (1973) when she said that:

> It is not that nursing lacks power but that nurses, operating against many opposing forces, have failed to recognise or use it to their professional advantage. (Ashley, 1973, p.637)

In case Ashley's research seems outdated, in 1993 Farmer opened her paper with the words:

> These are difficult times for nurses. Caught up in a political climate of oppression, there is a prevailing sense of hopelessness which is intensified by the absence of effective leadership of the discipline. (Farmer, 1993, p.33)

Farmer associates caring with good use of power in the caring relationships both to clients and fellow nurses. By virtue of not feeling empowered (Chapter 6) but on the contrary feeling fearful, nurses are encouraged to develop coping strategies which not only protect them but which are sanctioned by nurses as the "professional way" to behave. Some of the fears identified in this research were fears of getting nursing procedures wrong in the ward and getting reprimanded in public as well as getting `it' wrong and causing some calamity to the patient. This phenomenon supports Carlson-Catalano's (1992) assertion that nurses have a fear of getting `it' wrong and showing their vulnerability which might be used by peers to "put them down". And the **"IT" is often only known when the wrong is done**, so there is fear of not knowing what will be the right thing to do or say as this is only made known with the reprimand. This is particularly pertinent in interpersonal relationships where the norms are implicit and unspoken, hence the strategy of the `Professional Mask' (Jourard, 1971, p.178). This reminds me of a colleague who as part of my induction to a new job, said: "Just do what you think you should do and I will tell you when you are wrong". Such a culture encourages second guessing of `correct procedure' which the other holds as powerful knowledge.

The emergence of the `Professional shield' as a category was very dense and mainly manifested in the behaviour of the `Professional mask', to hide emotions and the fear of losing face (see figure 4.1, Chapter 4). This was the most significant strategy used in with-holding self as a strategy for self-management. The causes, attributes and consequences of the `Professional shield' were explained in detail in Chapter 6.

The mask makers I perceive to be those people who educate nurses in how to stay detached, who see role play in interpersonal skills training as "not real" and particularly those who actively encourage "role-playing" a role play (Pulsford 1983b) to further detach students from the immediacy of experiencing direct communication in an authentic intimate way (Berne 1972) with peers. The mask makers are those who actively encourage nurses into the socialised notion of "keep your head down", those who are fearful of confrontation, those who are unaware of the concept of intimacy in interpersonal relationships (op. cit., 1972) or who are aware and fear such intimacy themselves. To put on the professional mask is to engage in self-illusions about personal power. It occurs, I believe, when nurses use positional power with patients and junior nurses to enable them to feel empowered by having `power over' others. The professional shield, therefore, has two sides to it, the outer hard shell of the professional mask, of power over and `professionalism', and the vulnerable underside being shielded from the distress of the cultural milieu.

This summary of the research has aimed to draw all the strands of the research finding together to make a coherent conceptual framework without making the mistake of going back into analysing the data afresh, although the temptation to do so was strong. The following Sections give tentative indications of the consequence of this research to the three main areas of nursing most affected by the findings, that is, nurse education, nursing practice, and not least, nurses as people relating to each other within the different contexts of their work.

Consequences for the education of nurses

The key points which came out of this study can be placed under the broad headings:

- **Andragogical teaching of nurses in Higher Education**
- **The education of teachers in psychosocial theory and practice**

The educational curriculum advocated by Bevis (1989) based on a philosophy of caring, (as a personal quality) would be a model of human caring alive in the School of Nursing where nurses who had experienced caring for themselves, would more ably provide quality caring for their patients.

- **Andragogical teaching of nurses in Higher Education**

The education of tutors in psychosocial education and in andragogical educational approaches is an area which needs further exploration. The move of nurse education into higher education is potentially a consolidation of the traditional educational methods being applied to nursing, or `education from above'. Yet moving into higher education does not automatically imply the loss of the education of equals philosophically or methodologically. The education of equals was developed within University departments (Jarvis, 1986, Knowles, 1978, Heron, 1982, Boud, et. al., 1993 amongst others). My concern that nurses might believe that moving into Higher Education would force pre-determined teaching approaches on them was reinforced by Birchenall (1994). Speaking of teaching in Universities, he said:

> The nature of contact time with lecturers is more to do with the quality of interaction than with "wall-to-wall" teaching. Nurses would do well to heed this.

What is disturbing is nurse educators' perceptions of numerous undergraduate students coming into the educational institution once a year and being lectured to regardless of individual needs and preferences, and nurses imposing this same structure on student nurses. By doing this, nurses are reverting to the traditional education framework, abandoning much that is andragogical and individualistic about the autonomous learner and adopting a system of large groups receiving lectures in various subjects from psychology, nursing, sociology to biopathologies and psychopathologies. Any participative interpersonal skills training is moving back down the list of curricular priorities (as in practice it has always been, according to students in this study) with the same reasons given for this now in the 1990s as given in the post-war years up to the early 80s by nurses and tutors, that is, lack of space in the curriculum, lack of an assessment strategy for interpersonal psychosocial education and an attitude of "they will learn the psychosocial dimension on the wards anyway". The literature has been saying otherwise for years (see Chapter 1).

Most importantly, the need for congruence between what the educational philosophy espoused and what it practised needs to be addressed. Both tutors and students were found to be very dividend about the use of experiential learning methods for interpersonal skills training. In Chapter 4 some of the reasons for this were discussed. Often in reading about experiential learning the creation of the encounter in structured learning exercises seemed to be the main focus, whereas facilitating the other levels of learning are equally important and are implicit in the curriculum documents under the umbrella of reflective diaries, discussion of critical incidents, framing experience within a conceptual model already available, or creating a conceptual model to make sense of experience in action, and then applying the learning to nursing practice across different practice areas. The notion of learning to learn pro-actively and double loop learning (Argyris, 1964, 1976) are linked with the total experiential experience which are part of the ways of learning of the educated person. As an aside, the practice of games, particularly ice breakers and "let's pretend" role-play are only two of the many ways to access individuals' internal learning processes (Mulligan 1993b) in experiential learning, yet most of the research participants' perceptions of experiential learning and much of the nursing literature about experiential education (Kagan, et. al., 1986, Burnard,

1991) seem unnecessarily focused on the use of games and often, on the basis of whether they like games or not students will decide whether they will be actively involved in experiential learning. Andresen (1993, p.59) put it well when he says that teachers "often forget what it is to be ignorant and how they learned, therefore they have forgotten how to teach those who still have to learn". His remedy is to suggest that to teach, one needs to make the uncomfortable journey back to ignorance. This journey to levels of new learning can occur with experiential learning.

- **The education of teachers in psychosocial theory and practice**

Presently, nurse educators are already facing a dilemma regarding their teaching strategies and educational processes in teaching Project 2000 students. Nurse Lecturers I have spoken to in this last year are recounting tales of confusion in College of Nursing with large numbers of students coming into training *(50 to 60 at a time)*, and where the expertise to teach such numbers is inadequate even for discipline subjects where wall-to-wall lecturing is possible. However, teaching such numbers interpersonal skills training is virtually impossible. Many Colleges have established a small team of nurse teachers to teach psychosocial aspects of caring, and interpersonal relating. The teachers are often those who are interested in the subject and have experience through their training in psychiatric nursing or who are psychology graduates. These teams use "small group" work to teach such subjects as dying and bereavement, counselling skills, communication skills and so on; however, they are meeting the same "With-holding of self" with these students as was found in this study. Also these interpersonal skills training teams have access to these students for the Foundation Course only (the first eighteen months of a three year course) after which, nursing subject specialists, not necessarily trained in psychosocial caring or interpersonal relationship skills, are expected to integrate these subjects into the other branches of nurse training, that is, Acute Adult Nursing, Children's Nursing and so on. One of the problems nurse teachers in the interpersonal skills teams are speaking of is that now the "small groups" comprise fifteen to twenty students which is in fact a large group in "Groupwork" terms, and the same issues surround their management of groups as were found in this study.

Birchenall (1994) in the editorial "Striking the balance-a nurse teacher's dilemma" spoke of the need for high standards in the training of teachers. He went on to say:

> ... those who prefer to teach nursing must be properly prepared for their job, There is no place in the training and education of teachers for short cuts or quick fix courses,.. but they must be competent as teachers, which means being comfortable with groups of different sizes, teaching.students of varying abilities through a range of methods in an array of environments.

244

He went on to say:

> Under no circumstances should a teacher knowingly neglect his/ her students' educational needs because this only serves to undermine the confidence and respect which those who teach and those who learn must have for each other if the educational process is to be successful.

This, linked with Kagan's description of "the new and often threatening skills" (op cit., 1985, p.291) are important indicators that nurse teachers need to be educated in the Heron (1970) sense so that they know themselves intrapsychically, know their strengths and vulnerabilities, know how to manage their vulnerability educatively and know how and when they displace their distress unto others in their interpersonal relating. Being a psychology graduate or general nurse teacher is not enough to facilitate psychosocial education to a professional group learning about managing themselves while helping patients cope with illnesses, loss and bereavement. For the teacher, preparing for this form of education is an individual journey of personal exploration for the purpose of being a therapeutic agent for self and then for others. With Wilmot (1993) I would also advocate that nurse educators need to explore to what degree they feel free agents, that is, how they experience and practise self-agency in the Harré (1983) sense "to conceive of oneself as in possession of an ultimate power of decision and action". The argument is that to teach personal agency implies that one needs to have experiential knowledge of what such a concept means; know its boundaries, limitations and applications. If this knowledge is lacking then the ethical question, not unlike the one which instigated this study needs to be addressed, that is, what right has the teacher, teaching for professional practice, to teach what seems impossible to apply in professional practice? Beverley (1988, p.997) maintained that "it was untenable that the I-Thou values can be sustained within an institutional structure which is hierarchical". She speaks of double standards when trying to apply I-Thou philosophy with patients and yet "pull rank on a student or colleague". Her recommendation for nurses to learn the skills of being therapeutic with colleagues is through role-play, when in safety, as part of "play" they can analyse their performance. And here lies the main weakness in her argument: this research shows that nurses do not feel safe to role-play interpersonal relating with each other, even more so than feeling safe role playing nurse-patient scenes. My reflections on the phenomenon of emotional support is that change needs to happen from within, that nurses need to want to explore their interpersonal relationships for their own benefit and that the environment needs to be conducive to a very open experiential way of teaching, which leaves room for learning (Bevis 1989). But note that both need to be in place, willing participation by the learner is as important, if not more important, than environmental issues, and I put the facilitator's competence as part of the conducive environment.

The present imperfect situation in interpersonal relations identified in this study is not a good role-model for nurses. I believe, like Jourard (1971, pp.31-32) that it is still the person-as-self who plays the role and as such the roles should not be artificially separated unless there is known self-alienation. For nurse teachers, the skills of facilitating students making personal change must be with the student-as-self and not with the student as 'pretend other'. To do the latter is to encourage the split between the personal and the 'professional' and to be the mask-maker for professional practice rather than the educator of the person.

Consequences for nursing practice

Professional life events can be deemed to include: (1) physically and emotional staying and supporting other people through illness, trauma and pain; (2) managing medical moral and ethical dilemmas; confronting inadequate medical and nursing care; (3) being part of a working group and learning group whose specific focus is facilitating or learning to facilitate other people going through significant life events. It is to manage the complexity of this emotionally demanding work, I believe, that nurse education has embraced personal and interpersonal skills as part of nurse training, not just for the nurses' benefit, but to a greater extent, so that patients receive better 'emotionally distress-free' care from nurses. Distress-free care links with Heron's notion of "not projecting old hurt-laden agendas into current situations." (Heron 1992: 131-134). Distress-driven care links with Menzies' (1960) description of social defense mechanism against anxiety. Being distress-free does not mean suppressing emotions, rather it means that the nurse can be emotionally engaged, expressing sadness, joy or anger which is appropriate for the present situation s/he is encountering, but which is not laden with anxiety, fear or inappropriate glee which has its origin in past traumatic events. Yet, the nurse brings all of her past experiences, in the form of cognitive and feeling memories into every new situation. (Spinelli 1989, pp.8-9) The purpose of emotional education, in the form of self-awareness training, is to allow such memories to be surfaced in a relatively safe environment. This facilitates the individual's self-knowledge and acceptance, self-monitoring, self-correction and adaptation as appropriate, all necessary processes towards developing enabling (therapeutic) skills. The intention behind such self-awareness is that the nurse (or any therapeutic carer) can, according to Spinelli (1989, p.130) "bracket their own meanings and interpretations of the world so as not to make it their task to value, judge or criticize their client's experiences.. " when they engage in therapeutic interactions with their patients / clients.

The tentative question was asked in Chapter 1, whether the 'newer way' of working and learning was less anxiety provoking for nurses than in the years leading up to Menzies (1960) study. If not, where was the anxiety being displaced or how was it being managed? In this research, with the use of supporting literature, it was seen that the stresses on nurses are still very high and that nurses managed that stress by a variety of methods which could be summed up in the core category of 'With-holding self as a strategy for self-management'. The consequence for nursing practice is directly linked to education for practice. This education is not solely confined to what is on offer in the formal curriculum but in every opportunity the nurse takes to seek out knowledge and look for emotional support as a self-directed individual.

Wilmot (1993) spoke of agency and knowledge, seeing knowledge as power and as being either deterministic and reductionist where the learner has no influence. There is also knowledge which is liberating, which is inductive and multivariant and open to the influence of the learner. I believe that personal and professional knowledge has this latter quality when used and viewed by the reflective individual. To feel empowered the individual needs to perceive that he or she can influence events, create relevant knowledge, make decisions and take actions freely chosen, at the level of commitment if not at the procedural level. Notions of power as power-over others need to be part of an open agenda in assessing the ward working culture: comparing power balance with the ward philosophy of care and the ward educational philosophy with the intention of making these elements of interpersonal dynamics internally consistent, liberating and educative in the Deweyan sense (1938). Empowerment is fundamentally an individual state of mind, based on self-esteem (see Gregory 1994, Appendix F) and sufficient courage to assert individual rights and needs hence the need for nurses to acquire assertion skills. Having said that power as a force is individual, the force itself is dynamic and pervasive and can be channelled for either good or bad, depending on the intentions and influencing power of the empowered. For nurses aiming to empower patients via educational processes and Patient Charters, they themselves need to be familiar with the beliefs, values and practices which go to make up the empowered person.

However the reality is somewhat different. In Chapter 6, the category of 'Conforming to try to belong to the ward team' was discussed at some length. One of the results of that discussion and through continuing reflection as I write and read and speak to nurses during the closing phase of this research, is that the concept of "team" is misleading. Nurses use it, which is why I used it as a category, however, it might be more appropriate to think of nurses working on the ward as a working group rather than team nursing; it better defines the present reality as found in this research. Nurses aspire to be part of a team, this is based on their need to belong (see Chapter 4 and 6). Their expectations might change and be more realistic if they took on the notion of the work group, which has different connotations and fits more with the "Need for nurses to pull their weight" on the ward. Such 'pulling your weight' causes emotional stress and even exhaustion as nurses feel that they need to be seen to cope. Findings in this study support those of Smith (1992, p.14) particularly reflecting nurses' seeming inability to ask for emotional support for the stressful work they do, which some of them ascribed to a lack of team spirit which made it difficult for them to ask for help. In this study, nurses spoke of their interpersonal relationships as being more stressful than any exposure to patients'

247

illness. This is a difficult point to assess, as Menzies (1960) explained, and I agree with her explanation, that intrapsychic stress, which could be brought about by exposure to others' illness, dying and death, is projected out into interpersonal conflict where it is more easily managed. Rather than attempt to make recommendations to "get this right" as though there were a simple cause and effect chain which could be easily remedied, it would be more realistic to see the complexity of interpersonal relations as a matrix of relationships; intrapersonal and interpersonal, spanning emotional, cognitive, behavioural, intuitive and spiritual dimensions, with such underlying influences of power (personal and political), energy, perceptions, values and beliefs, within over-riding social, cultural and political dimensions. Seeking for single causes and simple solutions flies in the face of the epistemological approach used for this study so will not be attempted. However, Bond (1986), Mitchell (1988), Cole (1991) Smith (1992) and Dawkins (1992) are just some of the latest writers to focus on the emotional cost of nursing. Jourard (1971) and Heron (1982) would say that keeping emotions hidden, that is, putting on the professional mask, has a temporary effect of seemingly managing painful or stressful situations, however, the energy needed to repress stressful emotions creates more stress and dis-ease than the appropriate expression of feelings. This highlights the need for support for nurses whether they work in a designated "Intensive high stress area" or in ordinary ward situations. This study deliberately focused on work environment which would be accepted as the most common in a hospital environment, and as was seen, the levels of distress and stress among most of the nurses were very high. One of the unforeseen advantages of this study focusing on the average ward in terms of culture and specialism is that there is less reason for any distancing by hospital nurses from these findings. It is too easy, in my experience for nurses to say "Ah, but.." and "we are different or the situation is different", as a way of resisting personal change. In this they are no different from most people who resist change due to fear of the unknown or an `attachment for the status quo'. (Klein, 1976, p.98)

There is much talk now of changing the nature of support groups in some nursing units into group supervision in an attempt to remove the possible stigma that many nurses felt about needing `emotional support' for their work. From this research it would seem the support, even within supervision groups, should focus equally on helping nurses resolve interpersonal difficulties, managing the stresses of the work, and helping students and junior staff nurses particularly who may not have a supportive family to return to at the end of each shift.

Leadership issues and resistance to leaders had a part to play in the emergence of the theory in this thesis. It was not the focus of this study to look in any great depth at the organisational or managerial structures within which "enabling" interpersonal relationships needed to operate, partly because that is another whole study in itself as is the theme of therapeutic interpersonal relationships between the nurse and the patient (Chapter 3), and partly because it is difficult to perceive therapeutic relationships in a structure although it can be inferred from the behaviour of the relationships in a structure although it can be inferred from the behaviour of the people working within it. What can be discussed here is that the concept of shared purpose between the organisation, above ward level and within the hierarchy on the ward, and the individual seemed absent. Torbert (1978) talks of educating for shared purpose as being a neglected area of study. His argument is that working towards shared purpose will "encourage self-direction and quality work" (op cit., p.109), attributes espoused not only in the School of Nursing curriculum, but endorsed most ward managers.

How nurses can bring such `enabling skills' to their own interpersonal relations is based on the premise that if the nurse has internalised the concepts and precincts of the educated person, then he/ she will use them in relationships with all others, not just with patients. The strategies which ward managers use need to be congruent with those espoused in the School of Nursing curriculum, which within a humanistic approach would be normative-re-educative strategies (Chin & Benne, 1976, p.23). Here people's values and sociocultural values and beliefs are considered to be central to their wish and ability to make changes. Normative outlooks initiate change, therefore to effect change experiential learning is best as it accesses and encourages people to critically reflect on their beliefs and values, skills and significant re!ationships. Within the normative-re-educative strategies for change, learning in groups is powerful (Lewin 1951) for re-education.

The final word in this section goes to Farmer who says of nursing as a professional group:

> We have to find a way to help the "queen bees" in our discipline to recognise that power comes only through the empowerment of others. Fundamental to this is the promotion of caring in our discipline; only then can we fulfil our role in societies across the world. (Farmer, 1993, p.36)

A review of the methodology

In concluding this study, one of the two main joys I have is the knowledge I gained of grounded theory, the other is how I learned experientially to understand how to use it for myself in this research. This experience was both a joy and an agony for me at times. Coming from a strong constructivist stance (Chapter 2) in my beliefs and value system about the nature of being (of reality) and the nature of knowledge, it was important that there should be as little ideological conflict as possible while I studied such a large project. However, personal preference for a particular paradigm was not a good enough reason for choosing it. The research approach needed to fit the nature of the study, as well as the intended outcomes imagined. Within a constructivist paradigm, grounded theory was chosen (Chapter 2) as it best suited my wish to move through descriptive to interpretative work of social interactional encounters (May 1986). My strong belief in following the personal inner meanings approach based on symbolic interactionism, for the purpose of exploring deeper layers of individual meanings to understanding the social interactive processes at play as people bridged the gap between their inner (intrapsychic) world and the interpersonal world in which they engaged. As Glaser stated:

> The goal and key to grounded theory is that it generates theory that accounts for a pattern of behaviour which is relevant and problematic for those involved. (Glaser, 1978, p.93)

This was my purpose when I commenced this study and this purpose guided me throughout the data collecting, coding and analysis, literature study and the searching for the basic sociopsychological process (and problem) which motivated the research participants' behaviour.

The research started with a fairly clear focus, which was the interpersonal relationship dimension between nurse and nurse, whether tutor, staff nurse and student. As the unit of analysis, the research focused on their perceived and actual interpersonal relationships with each other. (Chapter 3) Forced comparison between tutors' perceptions of the relationships with students were not made to any great depth, rather patterns of meaning (Patton, 1990) which emerged were identified as being similar or dissimilar at a psychosocial level and were developed into theoretical interpretative categories of how nurses related to each other.

The data collecting comprised intensive interviews backed up by some observations, direct and indirect, and documentation in the form of hospital philosophy statements and curriculum documents. The advantages and disadvantages of the methods used were described in Chapters 2 and 3. However, here it would be useful to pause and reflect on two main gaps in the data sources, one being that ward managers (ward sisters in the research hospital) did not volunteer to be part of the study and the other being the paucity of the observational data.

The ward sisters in the general hospital were present when the senior nurse explained my research to them and the explanation came with an invitation to any sisters who wanted to be part of the study to contact me, and particularly the sisters of the wards on which I would do observations. The three sisters who gave me permission to do so seemed to take it for granted that, as one sister put it:

> If you want to know what they think and feel about each other, it would be best if I kept out of the way. Mostly I am at meetings so my relationship will be different.

I accepted this state of affairs without probing it too deeply, to have probed felt like an imposition and a demonstration of lack of respect for their right to opt out of intensive interviewing. I believe that this was a reasonable approach to take both ethically and methodologically. My reflection was that phenomenologically, in the work place, ward managers seemed to exclude themselves from the study of interpersonal relationships between nurses as they perceived that interpersonal meant 'social' and coming from a hierarchically higher position on the ward they did not see their relationship as 'social', but professional. They seemingly saw a difference between interpersonal relations and hierarchy which may account for some of the stress and conflict on the ward, which was discussed at length in Chapter 6. However, as a further study it would be very interesting to study ward managers perception of interpersonal relationships within this methodology, and would add to the many studies of the ward manager's role relating it to the psychosocial relationships they have with the ward work group.

The other main concern is the less than expected observational data. I had imagined being able to mix and mingle with nurses with some ease, so that I could in a sense be a fly on the wall as they related to each other in the clinical rooms, sluice rooms, dining rooms and during report sessions on the wards. This situation was discussed at some length in Chapter 3. However, I also need to acknowledge that I was very likely discounting the significance my presence might have had on the ward staff. Certainly for junior nurses to be told that "some researcher from a University is coming to see how you relate to each other" might have sent them all flying in the opposite direction. Permission for my presence was obtained from ward staff, to which they agreed. However, as a result of this study, I am not sure how empowered they felt to refuse, or whether within the functional-structural mode of operating of the professional shield / mask saying 'yes' to my presence, yet hiding from me at a sociopsychological level might have been culturally acceptable to the ward staff.

Also what I want to emphasise here is how my experience of feeling excluded in the ward is consistent with the findings of this study. If I had wanted to be accepted I, like the students, would have needed to get into uniform, rolled my sleeves up and worked like them. This need to be working to be accepted by the ward was highlighted most sharply in the many studies of the clinical teacher's role in the ward, (Kevern, 1987) This emphasises the importance given to physical work and yet begged the main question in the observations phase of this study, which was, What happens to nursing as a concept, when the physical work is done? This question has not been answered in this research, as that was not the focus. However, it may need some answers fairly soon, if the Minister of Health's recent pronouncements that the number of hospital beds will continue to fall drastically, as medical technology allows for more rapid key-hole surgery and shorter stays in hospital are realised. Will such highly technical environments need caring nurses, or technologists? Certainly for the surgery, technologists might be better, and nurses, what work will they do?

The complexity of grounded theory is that both the data collecting and data analysis are systematic strategies which need to run parallel to each other. Hence the use of sampling strategies is different. It was difficult in this study to convince myself that it was acceptable to choose a research site I knew, yet that was where the perceived problem emerged. Hence it was important to stay in the locality of the problem, rather than look for the same potential problem elsewhere. It was also difficult not knowing in advance how much data needed to be collected and from whom. My definition of purposeful intensive sampling which snowballed (Chapter 3) is an accurate one and it did help me to obtain data rich informants in a most effective and economical way. Its drawback was convincing myself that the whole method lent itself to `easy picking' that is, that any way of obtaining data was acceptable as long as it helped verify your emerging theory. Such thoughts demonstrated previous training in positivistic stratification sampling procedures for which I still hold a respect, but which were not useful for this study as they would pre-determine the sample and make impossible the need to be flexible to do theoretical sampling.

Reliability of the research finding was addressed by going back into the research field and checking my interpretations with informants, as well as with other nurses in different stages of the research. (Chapter 3) Using the strategies of constant comparative analysis and theoretical sampling ensured that the data `fit' and `worked' in the context they were found. The research finding was valid as those in the research field could recognise it as their experience of their interpersonal relationships and so endorsed my interpretation of, not only "What is going on here, but how?" (Becker, 1993, p.255). The credibility of the research lies in the integration of all the relevant elements to form a robust theory of a substantive type which is relevant and workable. The interlinking of the major sociopsychological categories, such as `Conforming to try to belong to the ward team', `Living the contradiction', and the `Professional shield' to the main basic sociopsychological process of `With-holding self as a strategy for self-management' is an individual choice with which another researcher could disagree. However, I was encouraged by Glaser's (1978, p.93) insistence that the choice must be made and that one or at the most two sociopsychological processes should be worked on at a time as the basic categories, basic in this sense meaning pervasive or fundamental patterns influencing behaviour. The notion of personal vulnerability as `Fearing intimacy' as a state of being was an important finding underlying the strategies people in the research used. To have identified strategies for self-protection without knowing why they might be needed would have weakened the emerging theory. However the combination of, `this is what is happening: `Fearing intimacy' and `this is how they (the informants) manage that': `With-holding self' is a sound integrated combination of the theoretical elements discovered in this research.

If nurses in general hospital wards continue to `With-hold self as a strategy for self-management', and as a consequence continue to give their own psychosocial needs and their patient's psychosocial needs least priority in the caring continuum, their ability to "come along side" patients and travel with them through their fears of illness, dependency, grief and loss will be at the very least naive and superficial, and at most detrimental to themselves and to their patients. For this reason, this research is important. It acts as yet another red flag, a warning, as many others referenced in this study and elsewhere have done, of the danger of people in the caring profession

252

not knowing how to create a caring environment for themselves. If nurses are being asked to manage other people's vulnerability, and they are, yet they cannot manage their own, then they are not good role models for junior peers coming into the profession nor to the patients or clients.

Looking forward

This last section looks forward to possible areas for further research arising from this study.

- A major question arose in the analysis of data which still needs to be answered: What is the investment for nurses (as a profession) in maintaining the status quo with respect to unsatisfactory interpersonal relations which seem to create a sense of dis-empowerment? Admittedly, there appears to be an answer in Menzies' (1960) account with reference to the need to put intrapsychic stress out as interpersonal conflict. However, from a Transactional Analysis perspective the intrapsychic conflict is explainable by Impasse Theory (Goulding & Goulding, 1979) which can be worked through on an individual level. It is individuals, both in education and on the wards that are the mask makers, or moulders, or mask breakers, showing new nurses how to be as a presence and in behaviour in order to belong. The question is, how this impasse can be addressed both individually and collectively in an educative way so that nurses can experience another way of being and relating to each other which is enabling.

- The second question springs from the many observations regarding the priority given to the interpersonal skills strand in nurse education and among student nurses. I believe that if the interpersonal skills training were given a new status in general nursing likened to that given in psychiatric nursing, then nurses and teachers would hold a different perspective on it. The training could be termed psychosocial principles and practice, psychosocial therapy in nursing. Assessments of knowledge and competence can be just as rigorous as other assessments (HPRG MSc 1993) so that nurses are as competent in psychosocial practice as they are in other areas of nursing.

- It would be very interesting to study ward managers perception of interpersonal relationships within a grounded theory methodology, and would add to the many studies of the ward managers role, this time relating it to the psychosocial relationships he/ she has with the ward work group.

253

Appendices

Appendix A

The College curriculum: the interpersonal skills strand

The College curriculum for the interpersonal skills strand was very comprehensive with the intention for students to be holistically educated in therapeutic interpersonal relating. The interpersonal skills strands is shown below:

Introductory Course:
- define effective communication
- define verbal and non-verbal communication
- develop listening skills, observation and
- interviewing skills
- define factors which enhance communication
- identify barriers to effective communication and ways in which they can be minimised
- Define the term "assertiveness"
- differentiate between "aggression" and "assertiveness"
- identify the components to the skill of assertion
- discuss ways in which criticism could be used constructively
- develop the acquisition of basic assertive techniques
- define stress and outline its effects
- identify methods of coping with stress.

In the six modules which made up the three year Registered General Nursing course the above topics were intended to be repeated in each module, each time relating them to either the patient in the surgical, medical, community, long-stay, acute and chronically ill category, to the elderly ill and the child and family where relevant.   Within the course, assessment of patients' need for counselling interventions were introduced in module 3. and application of basic counselling skills was introduced in module 4. (during the second year of training- see Appendix 1). The need to identify personal feelings and to be able to discuss them in the appropriate situation are written into module 2 and 5. Finally, in the 6th module (the last in their training at the end of the three years) the content is "Discuss the implications of working as a senior student nurse with reference to:

i) Power/Authority; (ii) Decision making; (iii) Communication;

(iv) Assertiveness

The new topics; Power/ Authority and Decision Making were seen as necessary in the final block to prepare nurses for the managerial responsibility of the trained nurse. Also communication and assertiveness from a managerial perspective seemed to be distinguished from other forms of communication and assertiveness. So throughout the curriculum the communication and interpersonal skills are clinical context related, however, whether these skills as personal qualities deepen either experientially or theoretically is not clear, either as an educational intention or in practice.

Appendix B

The analysis of data

This appendix is offered as a window into the analysis of data which was carried out in this research. It is an opportunity to illustrate the codified sets of propositions which were systematically drawn out of the data as described by Turner 1981 (see Chapter 2.) after Glaser and Strauss (1967). According to Harre & Secord (1972: 126), in ethnogenic social psychology, precision of meaning corresponds to accuracy of measurement in physical science. This concept is referred to by Lincoln and Guba (1989, p.242), within the constructivist approach when they speak of "stability" of data over time. This means that the data are dependable even with shifts of methodology and construction. The purpose of this appendix is to show how, within a grounded theory approach, attempts at precision of meaning were arrived at.

The intention is to present the first two interviews in some detail, (selecting nurses relationship with each other as the unit of analysis) to show open coding and theoretical memos, which although concepts already, will develop into more abstract concepts and categories (Strauss & Corbin 1990, p.72) that then directed the theoretical sampling in later data collection (op cit. p.207) (see 3. 8). The subsequent higher order conceptualisation is not shown in great detail, rather the substantive codes are clustered according to the relational dimensions and theoretical categories assigned to them as part of the constant comparative analysis. The more abstract categorisation formed the content of Chapters 4, 5, and 6.

The names of all interviewees are code names. The raw data are in the left hand column, open codes in the middle column and theoretical memos in the right hand column.

Interview with "Andy" - a student nurse

Andy was a second year student nurse training to become a Registered General Nurse (RGN). He had already spent about four months in the College of Nursing and fourteen months in various ward and community clinical placements. Andy was in his mid-twenties and had come into nursing having worked in more than one industrial job. The reasons for selecting Andy to illustrate coding were that I considered him to be "information rich". (Patton 1990, p.169) (see Chapter 3) Also Andy was the second person and the first student to be interviewed, therefore his interview data were subjected to line by line analysis and formed the basis of theoretical sampling. (Strauss & Corbin 1990, p.73) Andy called "a spade a spade" and was more than willing to share his opinions with me as "research is important in nursing" to use his words.

As this was the first student interview, I followed any leads offered which referred to relationships between him and all others who came into his world of work, leaving theoretical sampling until later interviews.

Extracts from data:	Open coding:	Theoretical memos:
JG. How long have you been in nursing?		
Andy. Just over one year and three months.		
JG. How is it going for you?		
Andy. Fine, I think, I've had no complaints..		Why does Andy accept no feedback from others as ok? Is this a feature of the working environment that students only know how others view their progress when they have done something wrong?
JG. .and because you've had no complaints, you think..?	1-positive self-assessment by absence of criticism from others	
Andy. I think I'm doing well.		
JG. and how are you with patients? Andy..Patients are often frightened and see others frightened.	2-awareness of fear behaviour in patients.	How useful is it for Andy to know others fears? How does Andy manage patients' fears? And his own?

260

Extracts from data:	Open coding:	Theoretical memos:
They might have a leg chopped off but they are still human beings, so don't mention the wound or injury, just be okay with them. Regardless of their condition they are still human beings.	3-denying of reality of mutilation. 4-separating out condition from the patient.	This separating out or "split" with the limb surgery, how indicative is this as a strategy for managing relationships? Does Andy's way of `avoiding patients' anxiety' reflect how he `avoids' feedback for senior nurses on the ward? and in the College too?

The interview discussed Andy's perception of his relationship with patients. This focused a great deal on keeping patients happy by saying little, getting on with the work, joking only with the cheerful patients and leaving the difficult patients alone. The next section of verbatim accounts refers to Andy's perception of his relationships with other nurses. To reduce volume, only the respondent's account is given unless it is essential to include interviewer's comments to show theoretical build.

Extracts from data:	Open coding:	Theoretical memos:
Andy- Life experience puts you in touch with people and you learn who to trust. My background was tough so you learn to be street wise, who to talk to and who not to talk to on the street. You learn to talk to all different kinds of people.	5-being street-wise:	Learning to know who is for you and who against you and to put on a "tough" front. Andy's background in `tough street' seems to still influence how he manages relationships at work. How does he rationalise about his abilities to manage his feelings?

Extracts from data:	Open coding:	Theoretical memos:
Inner confidence is what is needed. Good teacher might help with assertiveness, but you need the inner strength to express yourself to people. Inner strength is knowing who you are.	6-self confident 7-personalising toughness	Seeing inner qualities of independence as the main ingredient for communication.
With my work colleagues, I talk to them. I respect that they have got a job to do as I have. It's all inter-connected, like cogs in a machine, if one does not work it affects the others, so we should all work together	8-knowing self 9-being one of many-work gang.	Knowing himself in what way? The difference between personal self and social self. (Mead 1934) Does Andy have a strong personal self? It will be useful to see if the concept of self and self-esteem is a salient factor among nurses.
At work the machine does not work smoothly.	10-work-gang and pulled in many directions.	Being one of a team is recognised and the relational difficulties acknowledged. How does "not working together as a machine" manifest itself in the workplace? What are the consequences for interpersonal relationship?
In School, (S.O.N.1) you've got people coming from the bottom all the way to the top, from 'O' levels all the way to college level, and people like me, and people from the middle class families, and		
people with very little life experience. They have got a couple of 'O' levels and come straight into nursing, and others		A heterogeneous group brought together randomly for their three year training and

Extracts from data:	Open coding:	Theoretical memos:
who come in with lots of life experience.	11-being different, culturally/ socially/ educationally.	needing to work together quite closely for the duration of the course.
..and there is a lot of bitchiness around and people get two-faced. They have just left home where they were the centre of attention, and they come here to a different environment...		Andy perceives that the different educational / social backgrounds create complex dynamics with him and the rest of the learning group.
..so they try to get a group where they are still the centre of attention. They still want to be a leader.	12-life experience meaning work experience.	Identity crisis? Regressing to school experiences and behaviour, like school children? If so how does this affect their relationship together and with their course tutors?
The rest of the student group can either go with the flow of things, or they can take their own way, make others follow them or they don't have to be part of any group. You don't have to be friendly with the whole group (you started nursing with)	13-competing, inclusion/ exclusion in groups 14-re-creating what is familiar?	Adjusting to the social world of professional training. The insecurity of the new environment? Wanting to be in the 'in group'
On the ward, it's ok when the work goes smoothly. If they, (the staff) have a gripe	15-being insecure and needing recognition	Leadership issues are part of group life. Andy does not appear to welcome it or tolerate how the leadership

Extracts from data:	Open coding:	Theoretical memos:
against me, of a working nature, they shouldn't deal with this on the shop floor, it should be done outside. If anything happens on the ward, they should take you to one side, and say if they have a complaint, they should take you to the office and not in front of the patients.	16-leading and following in groups; belonging and distancing 17-selecting your friends & leaders	struggle is fought out, so withdraws? Deciding not to lead? To keep his distance? Andy has an awareness of group dynamics and seems to be able to decide for himself where he wants to be. Andy's opinions of relationships seem fixed by previous non professional job, influencing perceptions of instruction and team work?
They (the staff) should respect your feelings, so not stand out lecturing in the middle of the ward, giving out.	18-being respected 19-correcting is a private affair?	Andy does not want to be reprimanded in view of the patients, but in
Andy. You do this by staying as friendly as possible. Just keep talking down to a minimum, just do the job and if they (the staff) need a hand just give them a hand, ask them nicely for things.	20-respecting feelings important, that is, not being humiliated 21-projecting own fear of conflict onto patients?	Cover up the cracks in the professional facade? How does Andy conceal his feelings? What professional mask does he wear-humour and / or distancing? This supports Jourard's (1971) assertion that nurses as well as other professional carers wear a professional mask. How is such a mask made. who are the mask-makers? What are the properties of `mask wearing'?
They (patients) are relying on us to look after them, so you can imagine their worry about conflict among staff. They would say	22-covering up (the cracks in nurses relationships)	

Extracts from data:	Open coding:	Theoretical memos:
"God, if they can't look after each other (the staff) how are they going look after us?"	23-co-operating? Polite, distancing.	Seems important for nurses to present a united front for the patients' sake. Showing that you care for each other gives confidence to patients
Everyone wants others to be treated as they would like to be treated and the other way round.	24-seeing your incompetence? Seeing your vulnerability?	
Senior staff, I treat them with respect, because they have been in the job longer than me. They are in a position of authority over me so should be able to answer any questions I have.	25-asking for reciprocal caring 26-respecting authority	Does Andy think that nurses need to control (hide) their feelings so that patients will do the same?
They have got the ideas of what they can do in that job, therefore they should be able to	27-being `guided' or mentored by others as they "must know" 28-expecting much from the senior	No conflict acceptable for the patient's sake. Does this also apply to Andy as a learner moving from ward to ward? Andy seems to have a dependent attitude towards senior staff
You have no hope of saying what you think, so you give up and do what they tell you. It would be the best thing really. Do what you are told and get on with it to the best of your ability.	29-being confident depends on copetence of managers 30-seeing the need for change	Andy might be questioning their competence to look after him, (managerially) while he cares for the patients? Hierarchy of caring for carer?
JG-Is this an area of potential conflict?		Is Andy rationalising his with-holding of

Extracts from data:	Open coding:	Theoretical memos:
Andy-Yes. Don't stir the pan like, go by the book, without anyone getting hurt. The feelings I have about this, (ward tension) are best dealt with off the ward.	31-fearing rejection 32-being "put in his place" 33-keeping silence	suggestions to maintain personal distancing? Students best keep silent and do what they are told. Is this one of the problems of their learner status or transitional status on the ward, or both?
I go back to my room, have a drink, listen to music and so on. Most of the time I let (frustrating) incidents go by me, but if you've got people ganging up on you its best to ignore it unless its really serious or they are really hurting you in some way with what they are saying.	34-staying out of trouble 35-conforming 36-releasing tension on his own.	Andy avoids conflict at all cost? Maybe Andy had his fingers burnt before when trying to get what he wanted so now he is cautious and tense? Stifled communication at work. How does he share what is happening for him off duty?
It's no different from growing up and getting some people ganging up and it's ok. Growing up tough helps you not to take things too personally. Childish behaviour just bores me. basically you just make a joke of it.	37-brushing off or trivialising rejecting behaviour 38-deflecting personal attack	Is there a link between his silence and others not telling him how he is getting on at work? Trivialising: name-calling is "part of fabric of living with peers." The tough street syndrom.
In psychiatric nursing, they (the tutors) try to get the whole set together in a room and if you have anything to say, you just say it. You get the whole thing off your chest.	39-protecting self by labelling behaviour as childish? (trivialising?)	Managing interpersonal conflict by distancing or trivialising incidents unless they hurt too much.

Extracts from data:	Open coding:	Theoretical memos:
I have never seen that in General Nursing. There they say, "Well she (the student) is having a problem, let her see her tutor."	40-feeling `safe' to be honest about feelings/ opinions etc.	It is difficult to know whether Andy has become accustomed over the years to being "ganged up on". If he has, how has this influenced his behaviour with peers and patients?
Everybody keeps it (their problems) to themselves. Like a couple of lassies who started, really homesick, they asked the tutor if they could have a word, but the tutor did nothing. Like there is no team spirit.	41-silence and non-disclosing 42-problems should be solved by authority figures	In psychiatry, direct communication of interpersonal issues between students is encouraged to prepare students for the type of group work they will be doing in the psychiatric wards. The process allows surfacing of underlying interpersonal issues.
In our College set, you don't get any team spirit. Maybe on the wards there is more team spirit, they *(ward staff)* are all qualified, they have all worked together for some time. Students are there for a while, and they might get on well with them. But, like on the ward it's more of a close knit group, not like the groups in the set where you get so many differences.	43-holding back / closing down 44-belonging and not belonging	Is this a reflection of the cultural difference between psychiatric and the general nurses in the care of patients and in their training? Is it the nature of the work? or more historical influences, ie general nurses giving more priority to clinical tasks rather than the "understanding of the person" needed in psychiatric nursing?
There is a lack of trust in the school set, which is why there is not the support and openness	45-comparing transitional working	Some tutors seem to allow students to share problems, others do not.

Extracts from data:	Open coding:	Theoretical memos:
between the students	relations with permanent working relationships.	In the learning set, students come up against issues of bonding or not bonding in the only long term group they can identify with over the three years (outside their family).
JG. Lack of trust?		
The teacher is there to get a team spirit going and to gather people together to learn and work together, but it never happens.	46-being unsure whom to trust	
		Lack of common purpose?
		There seems to be difficulty with meeting individual needs and group goals. How is this tension managed by the learners and by the tutors?
There are just a couple (of teachers) for whom you have respect and the others don't stand a chance. They talk and their voices are monotonous or the subject is boring so students talk in the middle of the sessions. They will fool about with others in the room. You can have that many conversations going on that for the few who are trying to learn, can hardly hear the teacher speak. You don't have a lot of respect for those teachers.	47-not trusting each other in College	
	48-silence and distancing as a result of not trusting	Although this learning group formed 15 months previously, Andy sees it as being short-lived, whereas in fact his transient state is more obvious in the wards where he only stays for 6-8 weeks.
	49-vying for power and influence in the group	
	50-expecting conducive learning environment from the teacher	If Andy's experience in College is "like being back at school", which bores him, how does this get reflected in his behaviour? How does he learn to trust if he fears `being ganged up on'?
	51-needing to be controlled to learn?	
It's not easy to open up with a teacher, she is outside of the group, therefore you wouldn't open up so much.	52-needing tutor to be entertaining, or just keep the attention of the group?	Andy sees himself as "streetwise" and confident yet has difficulty relating to others in the learning

Extracts from data:	Open coding:	Theoretical memos:
You wouldn't open up to most of the people in the group, there are a couple of people who wouldn't mind, like me, the younger ones, who just talk	53-defining who is in charge	set, how are other students experiencing relating in the College of Nursing especially with
I don't like it (how the group works) but there is not a lot I can do..because if you try to organise things, everybody comes out with so many excuses it's unbelievable.	54-separating student from tutor status 57-selective sharing within the group	By 'opening up' meaning emotional and intellectually sharing.

What constitutes a large group? If the groups were smaller, would that make a difference to sharing and feeling part of something? Andy |
Some people like working in groups, some do, some don't.	58-splitting of group along lines of differences and size	does say that 'the younger ones' talk in small groups or are shy.
Some people try to get the group involved...but everybody has different tastes and you can't get the group together.	59-moving from learning group to social group with little success= maintaining distancing	Is the splitting of the group along competitiveness lines or emotionality? Is it preventable? How have these students been allowed to storm, and how do they 'know' what
JG. Socialising would help break down barriers and actually get people to co-operate?	60-feeling helpless	safety in a group means? How can the students disclose their ward difficulties from a personal perspective, if
Andy: Yes, but you get nowhere.	61-social bonding not seen as an option	they don't trust each. other?

Moving back to interpersonal relating in the ward, Andy's main concern seemed to be to minimise personal contact, to keep both patients and staff at a 'professional' distance. He goes on to say:

Extracts from data:	Open coding:	Theoretical memos:
JG. The part you said earlier, about communicating with patients, and being friendly with them, where do you see that linking with nurse education?		It will be important to check other students' perceptions of group learning and group dynamics.
	62-wearing the uniform equated with knowing your job	
Andy. Question is, trying to get everybody to teach it. Speaking to people is part of your job. They are individuals, they are here for a purpose, you are here for a purpose; to create an environment for them, because we have got uniforms, we should know better, like, if we have good communication and good relationships, like, they, the patients, are going to trust you. Everybody knows like, the more happy like, and contented the person is the quicker they are better.		The teachers asked to be confidence developers. The student wants to feel confidence in himself, even when he meets new situations. How might they do this? Qualities of reassurance and rapport seem important.
	63-engaging on a personal level	
		Interesting "should" and because they "should know" it's ok to fake it to give patients confidence. What about the ethics of this? and the nurses' confidence?
JG. Yes.	64-reacting on a personal level to critical patients	Teaching nurses to pretend, to put on the professional mask of competence?
Andy. The low of it is the psychological bit.. people worry about the slightest thing.	65-socialising away from the sick role	Dimensions of distancing between Andy and others (peers) and rejecting patients

Extracts from data:	Open coding:	Theoretical memos:
Patients need to have confidence in you. Even if you haven't got a clue what you are doing...	66-governed by authority	who reject him, yet being professional.
..if you have a difficult patient you could check what they are interested in... Try to meet them on a social level.	67-covering up ("wearing the professional mask")	Andy is likely to project his need of "being looked after" unto authority figures. This transferring of "parental responsibility" to
People in authority, Doctors and Sister should manage difficult patients to keep morale high.	68-giving as good as he gets.	authority figures is a feature of institutional living.
They can say "well you are not the only patient in the ward", so like put him down a bit.		To what extent is this part of the culture he is now in, or to what extent
The Sister, she is the captain of the ship, and she is there to make sure that things run smoothly. If she saw two conflicting sides, she is going to have to stop it, either by sending one of the people away or telling them to do the job and if they want to fight to fight outside. While they are on the ward, they do the job, and that is it, no matter what their personal grievances are.	69-needing authority figures on my side	is he bringing it from his past into the present and making the same demands for control and care?
	70-keeping the peace Sister acting referee	Andy does not seem to identify his need for skills in conflict management. His strategy seems one of with-drawing and letting others deal with difficult situations.
	71-putting down a `difficult' patient	Seeing management skills as something senior nurses need to manage students and
Because she has the authority she will have		patients.

271

Extracts from data:	Open coding:	Theoretical memos:
the skills (to manage conflict).		Conflict management not seen as part of managing self, or the peer relationship or the management of difficult situations with patients/ relatives.
Senior staff should be given training in managing conflict. I have seen some Sisters being able to do the job of nursing but when it comes to line management they can be useless at it.	72-assumptions that authority and competence should go together? 73-advocating authoritative control	Difficult to know why Andy thinks he needs to be a trained nurse before he empowers himself to manage interpersonal situations in College and on the ward.
JG. Teaching how to ask people properly, saying, `can you do this?. Using the right words. Andy-Yes. Management training would happen after qualifying as a nurse, because most people go through their training, qualify and just drop out. There is no point training them if they are going to drop out. JG-suppose it was part of your training as a student nurse, how to manage people and manage conflict so you can manage yourself and others?	74-knowing how to use authority benevolently 75-deciding who should learn how to manage conflict 76-dropping out- disassociated from `people skills'  77-dealing with one thing at a time  78-conflict management a `higher level skill' - not for student nurses	It could be that he can just manage one role at a time i.e. learner / junior focusing on "learning the ropes" in theory and practice and needs somebody else to "care-take his interpersonal needs" while he does that. Also the transient nature of his presence on the wards might also discourage him from much interpersonal relating. Finite energy may be used to 'get through the

272

Extracts from data:	Open coding:	Theoretical memos:
Andy-Well it would be fine, but there is not a lot you can do, if it is not part of your training. It would be relevant, well you might be in charge of a ward, where you need to be good (at managing conflict) but it should still wait until after the finals, (examinations) when people are going to be staying in the job.	79-linking self-awareness and assertiveness with management skills	day's work' and 'get through the training' rather than develop interpersonal skills. If this is the case, where is he getting the notion that interpersonal relating is less important than "basic nursing care".
	80-asserting seen as challenging "who is in charge".	
	81-fearing the undermining of confidence	
It is not ok that we don't have any management of people training as a student. I mean you can start off with self-awareness and assertiveness. But some people push it to the limits.	82-confusion about assertiveness and lack of co-operation	How does Andy separate out self-awareness and assertiveness training, which to him are relevant skills for students and conflict management?
	83-Seeing possible aggression as over assertion	
A helping relationship, what you find in the text books of nursing, being caring. When you come into nursing it's all about caring and looking after people.	84-assertive student seen as potentially more powerful interpersonally than authority figure.	
	85-Being in charge based on hierarchy not knowledge	Again highlighting discrepancies between seeing authority figures in uniform being able to control and manage conflict, yet an assertive student being able to undermine that.
	86-vying for power, feared or sought?	
I'd rather stick with the text book way and being friendly, like.	87-needing to protect the hierarchical position by exaggerating students potantial influence?	

Interview with "Lucy"- a Nurse Tutor

Lucy had been in nursing for 20 years. She was a specialist nurse and a qualified nurse teacher. Lucy's first interview was in two parts as she had a busy teaching schedule. She was also re-visited twice to discuss the emerging categories. Lucy was the second tutor I interviewed and this text is part of that first interview.

Much of Lucy's interview refers to the relationships between the nurse and the patient. This perspective is useful at an early stage in the research, as it reflects some of the assumptions, values and behaviours which are likely to infiltrate Lucy's teaching and her relationships with her students.

Extracts from data:	Open coding:	Theoretical memos:
JG-What to you are the most important aspects of nursing?		
Lucy- Well I think it is respecting people as individuals. Nurses need to be aware and understand the people they are caring for so that they can develop their potential. I make no distinction between patient and people, I talk about people.	1-respecting individuality 2-seeing uniqueness	Lucy aiming to respect uniqueness with regard to nursing care. Valuing of person is not role specific.
Nurses need to be aware of everybody around them , other health care professionals.	3-recognising that multi-disciplinary work is complex	Lucy realising her own and others' expectations are unrealistic when it comes to students' understanding of the significance of the multi-disciplinary team.
And part of that development is that the whole team needs to be in place so that you have senior people who can help newer people to develop.	4-developing a working relationship takes time 5-recognising the significance of senior 'mentors' in the	The need to gradually ease into the nursing role is seen as more facilitative for the learners. Lucy separates out the

274

Extracts from data:	Open coding:	Theoretical memos:
Lucy-I think that when you are performing in nursing roles, there needs to be times during the day, and even if you are counselling patients you are still the nurse, there needs to be a time when you just socialise.	nursing team 6-focusing on low level tasks, freeing attention to engage with patients? 7-meeting social needs-not in depth psychological needs	social care and links this with what students already bring to nursing, i.e. their general social skills. (Kagan (1985) speaks of this about interpersonal skills.) Socialising can be done while doing 'simple tasks' rather than when the nurse has finished working.
JG-When you say that your aims are the same, (towards patients and students).. and you		
JG-It seems from what you are saying that they (the nurses) build up an enabling relationship if they are more on a social equal level? Lucy-Yes, an equal level. I think that comes with time and experience. A lot depends on the type of previous experience they have had.. especially in education. JG-Do you mean if those experiences were enabling for them or not? Lucy-Yes,. They may have been disabling to some degree, (or) their	8-shifting between professional/ technical and social relationships 9-facilitating and enabling accepted as meaning the same process of helping patients get better 10-social bonding is facilitative	Enabling offered as a therapeutic concept as the term facilitation is often used in the College of Nursing as an educational process. Both words can mean the same concept in terms of intention. This will be interesting to explore. There is a need to see the difference between socially enabling and therapeutically enabling. Lucy is merging them at this stage. Creating positive inquiry skills and being able to influence what you learn and how you learn it,

Extracts from data:	Open coding:	Theoretical memos:
life experience may have been such that they have experienced being able to work freely and been able to be part of the decision making process then they will be more ready to being enabling for patients. Knowing themselves and having confidence in themselves, understanding themselves physically and psychologically. It can be painful to know your weaknesses. JG. You think that nurses need to know themselves before they can be enabling for others? Lucy. Yes..the nurse needs to know her own strengths and weaknesses. It can stop you being judgemental as you have got your own strengths and weaknesses that you would like to focus on, I guess.	11-carrying experiences from one stage of life to another 12-linking poor previous educational experience to personal and social development. 13-belief in self-exploration to make behavioural changes. 14-knowing yourself more helps you to be tolerant of others	gives confidence to relate to others? Lucy shows here her belief that self knowledge is an essential part of the enabling process for self and others. This links with the recommendation for self-awareness and interpersonal skills training in the nursing curricula. It also links with the pattern of teaching of these subjects, that is, moving from awareness raising to behavioural skills delevopment in experiential learning workshops. Seems that students need a conducive learning environment and that the tutor is directly involved with this. Lucy would want to role model enabling relationship by being particularly sensitive to why and how she confronts learners' lack of skills with relating to patients.

Extracts from data:	Open coding:	Theoretical memos:
JG-Right, say more about how you are with individuals then as a nurse educator? Do you see yourself having an enabling relationship with students? Lucy-Creating an enabling environment is very important. Yes, it always comes back to this; if you have a good learning environment that will enable new students to develop, then their skills can grow (so that) towards the end (of their training) they are acting as the enablers. JG-What part do you think you have, or want to play in developing skills of enabling in your learners? Lucy-I would want to be a role model and to give them time and opportunity to develop their skills. JG-How would you see yourself doing that? Lucy-It depends on the relationship, I would want to eventually move to confront poor	15-enabling skills seen as part of the educational relationship 16-creating an enabling environment seen as necessary in the ward setting 17-maintaining her facilitative role and including vicarious learning	Lucy's main aim is to maintain the rapport with the individual so that the channels of communication stay open and that the person does not feel so confronted that they withdraw their goodwill in the relationship. Do students have time to build up any form of rapport with the trained staff on the wards? When and how is it ok to give constructive feedback to students about their performance in a manner which will encourage them to remain open in disposition and ready to learn? Demanding change that the person is not committed too would back-fire. confronting challenges the person's self-esteem, particularly in the initial stages of learning.

Extract from data:	Open coding:	Theoretical memos
behaviour. It's getting to know them and finding the right time... JG-I'm wondering if the worry of offending the person can stop you challenging the disabling behaviour. Suppose you had a student who you found was really not being very enabling for the patient. What would you do?	18-Demanding change	It is difficult to know whether Lucy believes that people with very short-term relationships should not confront poor nursing skills, when most of the students are only on a ward for 6-8 weeks, and given the shift pattern and rotation to night duty, may only work under the same senior staff nurse/ Sister for about a quarter of the time.
Lucy-Each situation would be different. But it might be the way they are expressing themselves, then you do need to challenge them. JG-I am wondering what your thoughts are on how nurses are with each other, as opposed to how they are with patients? Lucy-We put labels on patients, and they are the target of care as are the relatives and participating in this is the student in enabling	19-delicate timing: there is a right time and a wrong time 20-concern for the student as a person and positive learning outcome	There is a difference between the teacher's ability to give constructive feedback and the students' willingness and ability to receive feedback. Both giver and receiver need appropriate skills for the interaction to work well. Lucy talks of her side only in this interview. Separating out who is the carer and the cared

Extracts from data:	Opening codes:	Theoretical memos:
and yet nurses are not enabling for each other. JG-Why do you think nurses do not support each other? Lucy-Some areas I have worked in are supportive. But it seems to me that the nurses are now more competitive with each other. the new grading system is helping that and it is value laden, what grade you are. It surprises me. The standards of care are actually declining. (End of the interview)	21-facilitating and confronting needs to be done with sensitivity 22-using professional judgement to inform when and how to confront 23-competing and being supportive are in opposition 24-nurses defending own position having less energy	for seems an important theme in the interpersonal dynamic among nurses. It would be useful to know if this was the case. Developing a grading system with payment awards has encouraged competition rather than co-operation? A culture is set up which makes potential rivals of peers. This was not the original intention of the grading system, so what has happened? Nurses needing to defend own position in the hierarchy? The system is a product of the culture which has been allowed to develop. What is the investment in maintaining this culture?

Theoretical constructs-taxonomies and categories

This section takes an analysis of the theoretical memos as axial coding to make connections between categories and their sub-categories (Strauss & Corbin 1990, p. 96) and to show the beginnings of a paradigm model, that is, relating the main events in the interaction to relational dimension uncovered by use of the six `C's (see Chapter 2). In Gregory (1994) diagrams are offered as visual representations of the categories to show how they link together. (Strauss & Corbin 1990, p.197) Theoretical codes and categories are linked into families according to the interrelated processes they address.   Diagramming is a way of showing which categories are related in a hierarchical way, that is, which category emerges as the core category and which are the sub-categories; properties of more abstract categories and so on. As explained in Chapter 2 (Stage 6) the core category should subsume and account for all the processes going on in the data between the group under study, although there may be more than one core category. Equally a core category may be a basic social process, which is what the researcher is constantly looking for in the analysis. According to Corbin, (1986) such diagramming facilitates an overview of the analysis and allows for greater manipulation of the data in a way that is impossible with memos.

The list below is an example of some of the many concepts identified in the first three interviews:

• Waiting to be told	•	Distancing self
• Keeping a distance from grief	•	Belonging to ward team / educational group)
• conforming / non-conforming	•	trusting / non-trusting
• disclosing / non-disclosing of self	•	supportive / non-supportive

Figure A-1 Indicators of the category: Facilitating personal learning

---

Antecedents (from tutor)

- allowing for uniqueness of the individual
- personal emotional support
- challenging disabling behaviour appropriately (supportive constructive feedback)
- mutual (tutors and learners) self disclosure of attitudes, values
- role-modelling intentional therapeutic behaviour
- need to have experience of facilitative role (links to **groupwork**)
- good understanding of group dynamics (links to **groupwork**)
- an educational philosophy which espouses personal learning is as important as professional training,

leads to:

Facilitating personal learning and development

Consequences:

- educational environment "psychologically" comfortable
- learners able to become more aware of the underlying group processes
- more able to risk-take in self-disclosure (with supportive feedback)

The above category **"Facilitating Personal Learning"** helped the development of the **Personal Psychological Learning Contract** which is discussed in Chapter 4. If this category, facilitating personal learning, is contrasted with what is stated to happen in some groupwork then the concept is a bi-polar construct with a negative pole of not accounting for the personal psychological needs of learners. These findings were discussed in Chapter 4.

The elements identified here bring together and form substantive codes into categories emerging from the first cluster of intensive interviews. Later category development was discussed in Chapter 4, 5 and 6. The concepts and main categories seemed to have fairly equal hierarchical status at this stage despite the efforts to place them into hierarchical categories. Further work needed to be done to look for attributes of the concepts, development of categories and identification of more substantive hierarchical order of main categories or one main category which could be assumed to be the overriding basic socio-psychological process (BSP) (Glaser, 1978) which this group of people are managing.

In summary, this appendix provides insight into the systematic breaking down of the data into manageable units of analysis for the purpose of uncovering the socio-psychological processes which are present in social interpersonal relationships, whether of a professional or personal nature. Understanding what these socio-psychological processes are and how they influence interpersonal behaviour is the mission of the grounded theorist. The above accounts giving embrionic conceptual maps are shown in their incomplete form to illustrate how such maps originated from participants verbatim data. Equally, it proved very difficult to present in a `tidy form' more complete category taxonomies as two dimensional drawings, for this reason, Chapters 4 and 6 provided more theoretical discussions than diagrams.

Appendix C

Structuring of time and interpersonal relationships

The concept of how people structure time is based on the premise that human beings have a stimulus hunger, which is a need for physical and emotional intimacy derived from the close bonding of the child in utero and infancy. This stimulus hunger transfers to recognition hunger as the very close physical intimacy is gradually diminished for the infant as it grows up and away from the parent. This need for recognition takes the form of physical handling, particularly in the young, to all forms of physical and social contact throughout life, even of the symbolic kind, with the hunger for positive recognition of being favoured, particularly from humans. The hunger is so primal, that in the absence of human recognition, recognition by proxy, animals, spiritualism, `fan-mail' will prevent the symptoms of sensory and emotional deprivation, or the shrivelled spine syndrome.(Berne 1946, p.14)

Berne defined `stroking' as the unit of recognition of one person to another with the stroking taking the form of any gesture, verbal or non-verbal that denotes recognition of the other's existence. Where the unit of recognition is responded to, that is, exchanged then social interaction has occurred. The premise is that any stroking (social interaction) is preferred to none, as the absence has profound biological and psychological consequences for the individual.

With the context of recognition hunger, there is structure hunger. That is how people manage their personal and interpersonal interactions through time as a continuum and using time to meet their recognition hunger.

Berne identified six ways or categories of how people use time, which will be only briefly described here for the purpose of offering a conceptual framework to illuminate the core sociopsychological process of **Fearing intimacy in the form of openness about self and honesty with others.** (Chapter 6)

282

Time structurings are: 1-Withdrawal; 2-Ritual; 3-Pastimes; 4-Activities;
                            5-Games; 6-Intimacy.

Withdrawal can be both a need for private time or a psychological withdrawal as a defensive strategy. Either way the only strokes a person can receive in withdrawal are self strokes, and there is minimal psychological risk of receiving 'rejection' strokes from others. It is in psychological withdrawing while still being physically present that the concept of 'With-holding self' makes conceptual sense.

Rituals are familiar social interactions (transactions) where the psychological risk, although higher than in withdrawal, is still very low. The interactions are 'safe' accepted social norms, such as mutual greetings, the 'proper way' to behave at business meetings and so on. Strokes are mutual and of a low risk factor in terms of 'getting it wrong' or fear of rejection.

Pastiming is less structured or pre-programmed, hence the individual has to invest more of himself / herself into the social transaction. Individuals' personal agenda is likely to be more foreground and the opportunities for both positive and negative strokes are higher. There is a greater psychological risk of rejection, but equally the possibility of more frequent and stronger strokes is present. The level of engagement is still superficial, (cocktail chat) as people who pastime, do just that, they talk about 'past times' without engaging with others to take action.

  Activities focus on 'here and now' communication, directed towards achieving some goal, solving a problem, as for example, my typing this Appendix is an activity. The level of 'recognition' in the form of strokes can be much higher than in the four previous time structuring modes, depending on the amount of involvement and directed energy the individual puts into the activity. Strokes may be conditionally positive or conditionally negative depending on the culture of the group, the competence of the individual in the activity (Stewart & Joines (1987, p.91), hence the psychological risk of rejection is higher.

Games These are psychological manoeuvres by which the individual seeks to get strokes through ulterior transactions. That is, the person has learned through experience that asking for positive strokes has resulted in rejection, ranging from minor to major rejection, so has learned to get recognised negatively. It is like the saying "bad press is better than no press". Games in this case are called 'psychological games' as they exist for the sole purpose of meeting the psychological needs of the individual. Games are a re-play of strategies from childhood which are no longer appropriate in adult life, but which the individual holds on to and plays out unconsciously as a way of still trying to get their childhood psychological needs met. Games are best understood when analysed within the framework of process communication developed by Berne and made popular in his book, Games People Play (1964). Games as a description is symbolic with the `distress-driven behaviour' spoken about by Heron (1989a)

Intimacy is authentic behaviour which responds appropriately to the immediate situation. There are "no secret messages, that is, the social level and the psychological level of communication are congruent". (Stewart & Joines (1987, p.93). Intimate communication is powerful enough to complete the transaction, leaving people satisfied that the issue has been resolved and resolved without manipulation, or other unproductive feelings or behaviour. Such intimate behaviour carries the highest risk of mis-understanding and other forms of apparent rejection, however the numbers of strokes both positive and negative are very high, so the reward for engaging in intimate communication is high.

When people cannot engage in intimate (authentic) communication they will often resort to games as the indirect way of obtaining strokes, usually of a negative type.

Bibliography

Adair,M. & Howell, P. (1989) 'The subjective side of power', in Hant, J. (ed) *Healing the Wounds-The promise of Ecofeminism*. Philadelphia, New Society Publishers.

Alexander, M. (1983) *Learning to Nurse: Integrating Theory and Practice*. Edinburgh, Churchill Livingstone.

Altschul, A. *(1978)* 'A Measure of Education'. Unpublished paper given at annual conference of the *Royal College of Nursing Association of Nursing Education, London*.

Altschul, A. *(1980)* 'Hints on maintaining patient-nurse interaction'. *Nursing Times*, 76 (15): 650-652.

Anderson, M. (1992) 'Letter to the editor'. *Nursing Times*, 88 (12): 14.

Andresen, L. (1993) 'On Becoming a Maker of teachers: journey down a long hall of mirrors', in Boud, D. Cohen, R. and Walker D. (eds), *Using Experience for Learning*. Society for Research into Higher Education. Buckingham, Open University Press.

Annett, J. (1969) *Feedback and Human Behaviour*. Harmondsworth. Penguin.

Antonovsky, A. (1979) *Health Stress and Coping*. San Francisco, Jossey-Bass.

Arac, J. (1988) *After Foucault: Humanistic Knowledge, Postmodern Challenges*. New Brunswick. Rutgers University Press.

Argyle M. (1969) *Social Interaction*. London, Tavistock Publications.

Argyle M. (1978) *The Psychology of Interpersonal Behaviour*. (3rd ed) Harmondsworth, Penguin.

Argyris C. (1964) *Integrating the Individual and the Organisation*. New York, J. Wiley and Sons.

Argyris C. (1976) *Increasing Leadership Effectiveness*. New York, J. Wiley & Sons.

Ashley J.A. (1973) *About Power in Nursing*. Nursing Outlook. 21, (10): 637-641.

Ashworth P. (1980) *Care to Communicate.* London, Royal College of Nursing.

Atwood J.R. and Hinds, P. (1986) Heuristic Heresy: Application of Reliability and Validity Criteria to Products of Grounded Theory. *WestBlackern Journal of Nursing Research.* 18, (2): 135-154.

Bales R.F. (1950) Interaction Process Analysis: A method for the study of small groups. Reading, Mass. Addison-Wesley.

Bandura A.A. (1977) *Social Learning Theory.* New Jersey, Prentis Hall.

Bannister D. and Fransella F (1986) Inquiring Man: The Psychology of Personal Constructs. (3rd Ed).London, Croom Helm.

Barber P. (1993) Developing the 'Person' of the Professional Carer. In *Nursing Practice and Health Care.* Ch. 14. Hinchliff S.M. et al (Eds) London, Edward Arnold.

Beardshaw V. (1981) Conscientious Objectors at Work. Mental Health Nurses-A Case Study. London. Social Audit Ltd.

Beattie A. (1987) Making a curriculum Work. In,Allen P. & Jolley A.P. *The Curriculum in Nurse Education.* Ch. 2.(Eds) London, Croom Helm.

Becker P. (1993) Common Pitfalls in Published Grounded Theory Research. In. *Qualitative Health Research,* 3 (2): 254-260.

Bendall E. (1971) The learning process in student nurses. Nursing Times Occasional Papers 1 & 2, 67: 43-44.

Bennis W. Benne K, & Chin R. (1976) The Planning of Change. London, Holt, Rinehart and Winston.

Benoliel J. *(1975) Research related to death and the dying in nursing research.* In Wilde V. *Journal of Advanced Nursing.* (1992), 17: 234-242.

Berger P and Luckmann T (1971*) The Social Construction of Reality.* London. Penguin University Books.

Berne E. (1961) *Transactional Analysis in Psychotherapy.A Systematic Individual and Group Psychotherapy.* London, Souvenir Press.

Berne E. (1964) *Games People Play: The Psychology of Human Relations.* London, Penguin Books.

Berne E. (1972) *What Do You Say After you Say Hello? The psychology of human destiny.* London. Transworld-Corgi Books.

Beverley K.H. (1988) Humanistic values and the ward environment. *Add-On Journal of Clinical Nursing.* 3. (27): 996-998.

Bevis E.M. (1982) *Curriculum Building in Nursing-A Process.* (3rd ed). St. Louis, C.V. Mosby.

Bevis E.M. (1989) Nursing curriculum a professional education: some underlying theoretical models. In Bevis E.M. & Watson J. *Towards a Caring Curriculum: A Pedagogy for Nursing.* New York, National League for Nursing. pp67-106.

Binnie A. (1984) *A Systematic Approach to Nursing Care.* The Open University Centre for Continuing Education. Milton Keynes, Open University Press.

Bion W.R. (1961) *Experience in Groups.* London, Tavistock.

Birchenall P. (1994) Striking the balance-a nurse teacher's dilemma. (Editorial). *Nurse Education Today.* 14, 1-2.

Black R & Mouton J. (1974) *The Managerial Grid.* Houston. Gulf.

Blumberg A. and Golembiewski E. (1976) *Learning and Changing in Groups.* Harmonsworth, Penguin.

Blumer H. (1969) *Symbolic Interactionism.* Englewood Cliffs, NJ. Prentice-Hall.

Bond M. (1986) *Stress and Self-Awareness: A Guide for Nurses.* Nursing Today Series. London, Heinemann Nursing.

Bond M. Kilty J. (1990) *Practical Methods of Dealing with Stress.* (2nd eds) Guildford. University of Surrey. Human Potential Resource Group.

Boud D., Keogh R and Walker D (1985) *Reflection: Turning Experience into Learning.* London, Kogan Page.

Boud D Cohen R. and Walker D (1993) *Using Experience for Learning.* Buckingham, The Society for Research into Higher Education (SRHE)Open University Press.

Bradby M. and Shoothill K (1993) From common foundation programme: recognising a status transition. *Nurse Education Today.* 13 (5): 362-368.

Brandes D. and Phillips H (1978*) Gamesters' Handbook.* London, Hutchinson.

Brandes D. (1982) *The Gamesters' Handbook Two.* London, Hutchinson.

Brown G.D. (1993) Accounting for Power: nurse teachers' and students perceptions of power in their relationship. *Nurse education Today.* 13: 111-120

Bruner J. (1960) *The Process of Education.* Cambridge Mass. Harvart University Press.

Bruner J. (1972*) The Relevance of Education.* London, Allen & Unwin.

Buber M. (1937) *I and thou.* Edinburgh: T & T Clark.

Burnard P. (1985) *Learning Human Skills: A Guide for Nurses.* London, Heinemann Nursing.

Burnard P. (1986) Encountering Adults. *Senior Nurse* 4 (4): 30-31.

Burnard P. and Morrison P. (1988) Nurses Perceptions of Their Interpersonal Skills: A Descriptive Study Using Six Category Intervention Analysis. *Nurse Education Today.* 8: 266-272.

Burnard P. 1989) *Teaching Interpersonal Skills.* London, Chapman and Hall.

Burnard P. and Morrison P. (1989) What is an interpersonally skilled person?: A repertory grid account of professional nurse's views. *Nurse Education Today.* 9: 384-391.

Burnard P. (1990) *Learning Human Skills: A Guide for Nurses.* (2nd ed) London, Heinemann Nursing.

Burnard P. (1991) *Experiential Learning In Action.* Aldershot, Avebury. Academic Publishing Group.

Butterworth T. (1984) The Future training of Psychiatric and General Nurses. *Nursing Times. 80* (36): 65-66.

Carkhuff R.R. (1971*) The Development of Human Resources.* New York, Holt, Rinehart & Winston.

Carlson-Catalano J. (1992) Empowering Nurses for Professional Practice. *Nursing Outlook.* 40, (3): 139-142.

Cassee E. (1975*)* Therapeutic behaviour, hospital culture and communication. In Cox & Mead (Eds) *A Sociology of Medical Practice.* Ch. 13. London, Macmillan.

Chenitz C. (1986) The Informal Interview. In, Chenitz W.C. & Swanson J.M. (Eds) *From Practice to Grounded Theory, Qualitative Research in Nursing. Ch. 7.* Menlo Park. Addison-Wesley.

Chenitz W. C. and Swanson, J. M. (1986) *From Practice to Grounded Theory, Qualitative Research in Nursing.* Menlo Park. Addison-Wesley.

Cherniss C. (1980) Professional Burnout in Human Service Organisations. New York. Praeger.

Chin R. and Benne K. (1976) General Strategies for Effecting Changes in Human Systems. In Bennis W G. et al. (Eds) *The Planning of Change.* Ch 1.2. London, Holt, Rinehart and Winston.

Clay T. (1986) Unity for Change? *Journal of Advanced Nursing* (1986), (11): 21-33.

Clay T. (1987) *Nurses: Power & Politics.* London. Heinemann Nursing.

Cole A. (1991) Stress: Pressure Point. *Nursing Times.* 87 (46): 24-28.

Coopersmith S. (1967) *The Antecedents of Self-esteem.* London W.H. Freeman.

Corbin J. (1986) Coding, Writing Memos and Diagramming. In Chenitz W.C. & Swanson J.M. (Eds) *From Practice to Grounded Theory, Qualitative Research in Nursing.* Ch. 9. Menlo Park. Addison-Wesley.

Corsaro W. (1980*)* Something old, something new: The importance of prior ethnography in the collection and analysis of audio-visual data. In Lincoln & Guba. (1985) *Naturalistic Inquiry.* London, Sage Publications.

Cowley S. (1991) A symbolic awareness context identified through a grounded theory study of health visiting. *Journal of Advanced Nursing: 16: 648-656.*

Davis F. (1973) The Martian and the Convert: Ontological Polarities in Social Research. In. Lofland J. & Lofland L. H. *Analysing Social Settings: A Guide to Qualitative Observation and Analysis.* (2nd ed). Belmont. Wadsworth Publishing Company.

Davis M. (1986) Observation in Natural Settings. In Chenitz W.C. & Swanson J.M. *From Practice to Grounded Theory, Qualitative Research in Nursing.* Ch. 5. Menlo Park. Addison-Wesley.

Dawkins C. (1992) Ditching the Professional face. *Nursing Standards. 7,* (23): 50.

Denzin N.K. (1978) *The Research Act: A Theoretical Introduction to Sociological Methods.* New York. McGraw-Hill.

Denzin N.K. (1984) *On Understanding Emotions.* Social and Behavioural Science Series. San Francisco. Jossey-Bass.

Denzin N.K. (1989) *Interpretive Biography.* Qualitative Research Series. No. 17. London, Sage Publications.

Department for Education (1991) *The Parents' Charter.* Department for Education London, HMSO.

Deurzen-Smith E. van (1988) *Existential Counselling in Practice.* London, Sage Publications.

Deutsch, M. (1973) *The Resolution of Conflict-constructive and destructive processes.* New Haven, New York Press.

Dewey J. (1916) *Education and Democracy.* New York. The Free Press.

Dewey J. (1938) *Experience and Education.* New York. Macmillan Publishing Company.

Douglas T. (1983) *Groups. Understanding people gathered together.* London. Tavistock Publications.

Dunlop F. (1984) *The Education of Feeling and Emotion.* U.K. George Allen & Unwin.

Egan G. (1982) *The Skilled Helper: Models Skills and Methods for Effective Helping.* (2nd.ed). Monterey. Brooks/ Cole Publishing Company.

Egan G. (1986) *The Skilled Helper: A Systematic Approach to Effective Helping.* 2st. Ed. Monterey. Brooks/ Cole Publishing Company.

Elden M. (1981) Sharing the research work: participative research and its role demands. In Reason P. & Rowan J.(eds) *Human Inquiry: A sourcebook of new paradigm research.* Ch. 22. Chichester. John Wiley & Sons.

Ellis A. (1973) *Humanistic Psychotherapy: The Rational Emotive Approach.* New York: Julian Press.

English National Board.(1987) *Managing Change in Nurse Education.* London. The English National Board for Nursing, Midwifery and Health Visiting.

English National Board (1990) Devolved continuous assessment for courses leading to Parts 1, 3, 5, 8, 12, 13, 14 and 15 of the professional register. *English National Board for Nursing, Midwifery and Health Visiting.* London.

Evans C. (1978) *Psychology: A Dictionary of the Mind, Brain and Behaviour.* London. Arrow Books.

Evers H (1984) *Patients' Experiences and Social Relations in Geriatric Wards.* (unpublished PhD thesis: University of Warwick.

Fagerhaugh S. (1986) Analyzing data for basic social processes. In Chenitz W.C. & Swanson J.M. (Eds) *From Practice to Grounded Theory: Qualitative Research in Nursing.* Ch. 11. Menlo Park. Addison-Wesley.

Farmer B. (1993) The use and abuse of power in nursing. *Nursing Standard. Clinical Ethics (23)* February 24th, (7): 33-36

Faulkner A. (1980) *The Student Nurses' Role in Giving Information to Patients.* Aberdeen Unpublished MLitt thesis, Aberdeen University.

Faulkner A Bridge W. and Macleod Clark J. (1983) *Teaching Communication in Schools of Nursing: A survey of Directors of Nurse Education.* Paper given at RCN Conference. Brighton.

Field P.A. and Morse J.M (1985) *Nursing Research: The Application of Qualitative Approaches.* London. Croom Helm.

Fielding R.and Llewelyn S.P. (1987) Communication training in nursing can damage your health and enthusiasm: some warnings. *Journal Of Advanced Nursing* 12: 281-290.

Firth J., McIntee J., McKeown P. and Britton P. (1986) Interpersonal support amongst nurses at work. *Journal of Advanced Nursing.* 11: 273-282.

Freire P. (1972) *Pedagogy of the Oppressed.* Harmonsworth. Penguin.

Fretwell J.E. (1978) *Socialisation of Nurses: Teaching and Learning in Hospital Wards.* Unpublished PhD thesis. Warwick University. England.

Fretwell J.E. (1980) An Inquiry into the Ward Learning Environment *Nursing Times. Occasional Paper.* 76, No. 16.

Fretwell J.E. (1982) *Ward Teaching and Learning.* London. The Royal College of Nursing.

General Nursing Council. (1977) *Educational Policy 1977. Circular 77/19 A-D* GNC. London.

General Nursing Council (1982) Training Syllabus-Register of Nursing-Mental Health. London. GNC.

Gibbs G. (1992) *Improving the quality of student learning.* Bristol. Technical and educational Services.

Gijbels H. (1993) Interpersonal skills training in nurse education: Some theoretical and curricular considerations. *Nurse Education Today. 13.* 458-465.

Glaser B.G. and Strauss A.L (1965) *Awareness of Dying.* Chicago. Aldine Publishing CO.

Glaser B.G. and Strauss A.L. (1967) *The Discovery of Grounded Theory: Strategies for Qualitative Research.*Chicago, Aldine Publishing Company.

Glaser B.G. and Strauss A.L (1968) *Time for Dying.* Chicago. Aldine Publishing Company.

Glaser B.G. (1978) *Theoretical Sensitivity: Advances in the Methodology of Grounded Theory.* Mill Valley, California. The Sociology Press.

Gordon T. (1977) *Leadership Effectiveness Training.* Westminster, USA. Wyden Books. McKay Publishers.

Gott, M. (1982) Theories of Learning and the Teaching of Nursing. *Nursing Times Occasional Paper* 78, (11): 41-44

Goulding M.M. and Goulding R.L. *(1979)* *Changing Lives Through Re-decision Therapy.* New York. Brunner/Mazel Inc.

Gow M. (1983) *How Nurses' Emotions Affect Patient Care: Self-Studies by Nurses.* New York. Springer Publication Company.

Graham H. (1983) Caring: a labour of love, in Finch J. & Groves D. (eds) *A Labour of Love: Women, Work and Caring.* London. Routledge and Kegan Paul.

Graham R.J. ((1981)) Understanding the benefits of poor communication. *Interface* 11: 80-82.

Gregory J.M. (1993) *Continuing Professional Development Courses Brochure* Guildford. University of Surrey. Human Potential Resource Group.

Gregory J M (1994) *A Grounded Theory Study of the Education of Hospital Nurses: How Education for Interpersonal Relating Influcences the Way Nurses Relte to Each Other in the College and on the Ward.* (unpublished PhD Thesis: Guildford, Unversity of Surrey)

Guba E.G. and Lincolm Y.S. (1989) *Fourth Generation Evaluation.* London. Sage Publication.

Guppy A. (1991) Job satisfaction and occupational stress in UK general hospital nursing staff. In *Work-and-Stress.* Oct-Dec Vol 5(4): 315-323.

Hall J. (1982) *Psychology for Nurses and Health Visitors.* London. The British Psychological Society and Macmillan Press Ltd.

Hammersley M.and Atkinson P. (1983) *Ethnography, Principles in Practice.* London. Tavistock Publications.

Hanson P. (1973) "The Johari Window: A Model for soliciting and giving feedback" In Pfeiffer & Jones. *Annual Handbook for Group Facilitators.* University Associates.

Harmer B. and Henderson V. (1955) *Textbook of the Principles and Practices of Nursing.* (5th. Ed). New York. Macmillan Inc.

Harré R. and Secord P.F. (1972) *The Explanation of Social Behaviour.* Oxford. Basil Blackwell.

Harré R. (1983) *Personal Being.* Oxford, Basil Blackwell.

Harris T.A. (1973) *I'm OK-Your OK.* London, Pan Books.

Hawkins P. and Shohet R. (1989) *Supervision in the Helping Professions.* Milton keynes. Open, University Press.

Hayward (1975) *Information: A prescription Against Pain* London. Royal College of Nursing.

Hayman B. and Shaw M. (1984) Looking at relationships in nursing. Skevington S. (Ed) In *Understanding Nurses-The Social Psychology of Nursing.* Ch.2. John Wiley & Sons Ltd. Chichester.

Heron J. (1974) *The Concept of a Peer Learning Community.* Guildford. University of Surrey, Human Potential Research Project.

Heron J. (1977a) *Catharsis in Human Development.* Guildford. The University of Surrey, The Human Potential Research Project.

Heron J. (1977b) *Behavioural Analysis in Education and Training.* London/ Guildford. British Postgraduate Medical Federation and the University of Surrey. Human Potential Research Group.

Heron J. (1977c) *Dimensions of Facilitator Styles.* Guildford, University of Surrey, Human Potential Research Project.

Heron J (1981) Philosophical basis for a new paradigm. In Reason P. & Rowan J. *Human Inquiry, a sourcebook of new paradigm research.* Ch.2. Chichester. John Wiley & Sons.

Heron J. (1982) *Education of the Affect.* Guildford. University of Surrey. Human Potential Research Project.

Heron J. (1989)a *The Facilitators' Handbook.* London. Kogan Page.

Heron J. (1989)b *Six Category Intervention Analysis.* (3rd ed). Guildford. University of Surrey, Human Potential Resource Group.

Heron J. (1990) *Helping The Client: A creative practical Guide.* London. Sage Publication.

Heron J. (1992) *Feeling and Personhood. Psychology in Another Key.* London. Sage Publication.

Heron J. (1993) *Group Facilitation: Theories and Models for Practice.* London. Nicols/ GP Publishing. Kogan Page.

HMSO (1966) Report of the Committee on Senior Nursing Staff Structure. London. *Ministry of Health Scottish Home and Health Department.* "Salmon Report" HMSO.

HMSO (1991) *Citizen's Charter (CM 1599).* London. HMSO.

HMSO (1989) *Working for Patients. The Health Service Caring for the 90's.* Cmd 555) London. HMSO.

HMSO (1993/4) *Maladministration and redress.* London. Houses of Commons Paper 504-ii. Select Committee on the Parliamentary Commissioner for Administration. HMSO.

Hockey L. (1976) *Women in Nursing.* London. Hodder & Stoughton.

Holden R. (1991) Responsibility and autonomous nursing practice. *Journal of Advanced Nursing.* 16 (4): 398-403.

Hopson B. and Scally M. ((1981)) *Lifeskills Teaching.* (U.K.) McGraw Hill Co.

House R.J. and Rizzo J.R. (1972) Role conflict and ambiguity as critical variables in a model of organisational behaviour. *Organisational Behaviour and Human Performance.* 7: 467-505.

Hoy R.A., Moustafa A.H. and Skeath A. (1986) *Balancing the Nurse Curriculum.* Tunbridge Wells, Costello.

Human Potential Resource Group. (1993) *MSc. in Change Agent Skills and Strategies.* Course Handbook, Section5. Unpublished Student Guide. Guildford. University of Surrey. Human Potential Resource Group.

292

Hutchinson S. (1986) Grounded Theory: The Method. In Munhall P. & Oiler C.J. *Nursing Research. A Qualitative Approach.* Ch.6. Connecticut. Appleton-Century- Crofts/Norwalk.

James N. (1989) 'Emotional labour, skills and work in the social regulation of feelings'. *The Sociological Review,* 37, (1): 15-42.

James V. (1986) *Dare and Work in Nursing the Dying.* PhD Thesis: University of Aberdeen.

Jaques D. (1991) *Learning In Groups.* 2nd. Ed. London. Kogan Page.

Jarvis P. (1985) *The Sociology of Adult and Continuing Education.* London. Croom Helm.

Jarvis P. (1986) Janforum-Nurse Education and Adult Education: a question of the person. *Journal of Advanced Nursing.* 11: 465-469

Jarvis P. (1992) Paradoxes of Learning in Late Modernity. *ACACE* Anahein. Unpublished Paper. Guildford. University of Surrey. Dept of Educational Studies.

Johnson D W. (1990) *Reaching Out: Interpersonal Effectiveness and Self-Actualisation.* (4th ed). Englewood Cliffs, N.I. Prentice Hall.

Jourard S. (1971) *The Transparent Self.* New York. van Nostrand Reinhold Company Inc.

Jung C.G. (1971) *The Portable Jung.* (Ed,.J. Cambell) New York. The Viking Press.

Jung C. G. (1977) Psychological Types. In *Collected Works,* Vol. 6. Princeton: Princeton University Press.

Jupp V.and Miller P. (1980) Glossary. *Research Methods in Education and the Social Sciences.* DE304.G. Milton Keynes. Open University. The Open University Press.

Kagan C. (1985) *Interpersonal Skills in Nursing-Research and Application.* Kagan editor. London. Croom Helm.

Kagan C., Evans J.and Kay B. (1986) *A Manual of Interpersonal Skills for Nurses - anExperiential Approach.* Lippincott Nursing Series. London. Harper & Row.

Kalish B. (1973) What is Empathy. American Journal of Nursing 73: 1548-1552.

Kalisch P. *(1971)* Strategies for Developing Nurse Empathy. *Nursing Outlook,* 19: 14-718.

Kalpin A. (1964) *The Conduct of Inquiry: Methodology for Behavioural Science.* Scranton. Pennsylvania. Chandler Publishing.

Kelly G.A. (1955) *The Psychology of Personal Constructs.* Vols 1 & 2. New York. Norton.

Kilty J. (1978) *Self and Peer Assessment.* Guildford. University of Surrey. Human Potential Research Project.

Kincey J. & Kat B. (1984) How can nurses use social psychology to study themselves and their roles? In Skevington S. (Ed) *Understanding Nurses-*

The Social Psychology of Nursing. Ch. 1. Chichester. John Wiley & Sons Ltd.

King I.M. (1971) *Towards a Theory of Nursing.* New York: John Wiley.

Klein D. (1976) Some Notes on the Dynamics of Resistance to Change: The Defender Role. In. Bennis W G. et al. *The Planning of Change.* Ch 3.2. USA. Holt, Rinehart and Winston.

Knowles M. (1972) *The Modern Practice of Adult Education: Andragogy versus Pedagogy.* New York. Associated Press.

Knowles M. (1978) *The Adult Learner-A Neglected Species.* (2nd Ed) Houston. Gulf.

Kobasa S. C. (1982) Hardiness and Health: A Prospective Study. *Journal of Personality and Social Psychology.* (1982), 42, (1): 168-177

Kohler W. (1970) *Gestalt Psychology: An Introduction to New Concepts in Modern Psychology.* New York. Liveright.

Kolb D. A. (1984) *Experiential Learning-Experience as the Source of Learning and Development.* London. Prentice-Hall.

Koldjeski D. (1990) Towards a Theory of Professional Nursing Caring: A Unified perspective. In Leininger M. & Watson J. (Eds) *The Caring Imperative In Education.* Chapter 4. New York. Centre for Human Caring. National League for Nursing.

Kratz C. (1980) *The Nursing Process.* (3rd edition) London. Bailliere Tindell.

Kratz C. (1984) Minorities and Power. *Lampada.* No. 1. August (1984).

Laing R.D. (1965) *The Divided Self.* Harmondsworth. Penquine Books.

Laing R.D. (1972) *Knots.* Harmmonsworth. Penguin.

Lalljee M. (1976) *Social Psychology.* D305. Social Interaction-Block 12. Part 1. Milton Keynes The Open University Press.

La Monica E. (1976) Empathy training as the major trust of a staff development programme. *Nursing Research.* 25, (6): 447-451.

Lancaster, A. (1972) *Nurse Teacher-the report of an opinion survey.* London. Churchill Livingstone,

Lathlean J. and Farnish S. (1984) The Ward Sister Training Project; an evaluation of a training scheme for ward sisters. London. *Nursing Education Research Unit.* Chelsea College, University of London.

Learn C. D. (1990) The Moral Dimension: Humanism in Education in The Caring Imperative. In Leininger M. Watson J. (eds) *The Caring Imperative in Education.* Ch.21. New York. Centre for Human Caring. National League for Nursing.

Leininger M. (1985) *Qualitative Research Methods in Nursing.* (Ed) Philadelphia. W.B. Saunders Company Inc.

Leininger M. and Watson J. (Eds) (1990) *The Caring Imperative in Education.* New York. Centre for Human Caring. National League for Nursing.

Lewin K. (1951) *Field Theory in Social Sciences.* New York. Harper & Row.

Ley P. (1972) Complaints made by hospital staff and patients, a review of the literature. *Bulletin of the British Psychological Society.* 25. 115-120

Ley P. (1982) Satisfaction, compliance and communication. *British Journal of Clinical Psychology. 31,* 241-245.

Light R. & Pillemer D. (1982) Numbers and Narrative: Combining their strength in research reviews. In Munhall & Oiler (1986) *Nursing Research. A Qualitative Perspective.* Connecticut. Appleton-Century-Crofts/ Norwalk.

Lincoln Y.S. and Guba E.G. (1985) *Naturalistic Inquiry.* London. Sage Publications.

Lincoln Y.S and Guba E.G. (1989) *Fourth Generation Evaluation.* London. Sage Publications.

Lindop E. (1989) Individual stress and its relationship to termination of nurse training. *Nurse Education Today.* 9, 172-179.

Llewelyn S.P. (1984) The Cost of Giving: emotional growth and emotional stress. In Skevington S, (Ed) *Understanding Nursing-The Social Psychology of Nurses.* (1984) Ch. 3. Chichester. John Wiley & Sons Ltd.

Lofland J. and Lofland L. H. (1984) *Analysing Social Settings: A Guide to Qualitative Observation and Analysis.* (2nd ed). Belmont. Wadsworth Publishing Company

Luft J. and Ingram H. (1967) *Of Human Interaction: The Johari Model.* Mayfield, Palo Alto,

Lutzen K. (1990) Moral sensing and ideological conflict. Aspects of the therapeutic relationship in psychiatric nursing. *Scandinavian Journal of Caring Science.* 4(2): 69-76.

Macleod-Clark J. (1982) *"Nurse-patient Verbal Interaction",* Unpublished PhD thesis. University of London

Macleod- Clark J. (1985) The Development of Research in Interpersonal Skills in Nursing. In Kagan C, (ed) *Interpersonal Skills in Nursing: Research and Application.* London. Croom Helm.

MacMurray J. 1935 *Reason and Emotion.* London. Faber.

Maguire P. (1985) Consequences of poor communication between nurses and patients. In *Nursing.* 2. (38): 1115-1118

Marshall J. (1980) Stress amongst nurses. In Cooper C.L. & Marshall J. (eds). *White Collar and Professional Stress.* New York. Wiley.

Marson S.N. (1985) *Personal and Professional Development.* Sheffield. National Health Services. Learning Resources Unit.

Maslow, A.H. (1970) *Motivation and Personality.* 2nd Ed. New York. Harper.

Maslow A.H. (1972) "Defence and Growth" In M.L. Silberman, J.S. Allender and J.M. Yanoff: *The Psychology of Open Teaching and Learning.* Boston. Little Brown.

May K.A. (1986) Writing and evaluating the grounded theory research approach. In Chenitz W.C. & Swanson J.M. (Eds) *From Practice to*

Grounded Theory, Qualitative Research in Nursing. Ch.12. Menlo Park. Addison-Wesley Publishing Company.

McGuire W. and Hull R.F.C. (1977) *C.G.Jung Speaking:Interviews and Encounters.* Picardo USA. Pan Books.

McKay M. and Fanning P. (1987) *Self Esteem.* Oakland, New Harbinger Publications

Mead G.H. (1934) Mind, Self and Society. Chicago. Chicago University Press.

Melia K. (1987) *Learning and Working: The Occupational Socialisation of Nurses.* London. Tavistock Publications Ltd.

Menzies, I.E.P. (1960) 'A case study in the functioning of a social system as a defence against anxiety' *Human Relations.* 13:95-121 Reprinted as Tavistock Pamphlet 3 (1970)

Miles M. (1981) Learning to work in Groups: A Programme Guide for Educational Leaders. In. Jaques D. (1991) *Learning In Groups.* 2nd. Ed. London. Published by Kogan Page.

Minardi H.A. and Riley M (1988) Providing psychological safety through skilled communication. *Nursing; The Add-On Journal of Clinical Nursing-*Third series-27: 990-992.

Misiak H.and Sexton V.S. (1973) *Penomenological, Existential and Humanistic Psychologies: A Historical Survey.* New York. Grune and Stratton.

Mitchell R.G. (1988) The Emotional Cost of Nursing. *Nursing: The Add-on Journal of Clinical Nursing.* Third series-28:1021-1025.

Moores B. and Moult A (1979) The relationship between the level of nurse staffing and the pattern of patient care and staff activity. *Journal of Advanced Nursing.* 4. 299-306.

Moores B. and Thompson A.(1975) Attitude to student nurses allocation programmes, *International Journal of Nursing Studies.* 12. 107-117.

Moscovici S. and Lage E. (1976) Studies in Social Influence: III. Majority versus minority influence in a group. *European Journal of Social Psychology 6,* 149-74.

Mulligan J. (1993a) *Module 2-Understanding Personal Development.* Unpublished MSc module for the MSc in Change Agent Skills and Strategies. Guildford. University of Surrey, Human Potential Resource Group.

Mulligan J. (1993b) Activating Internal Learning Processes in Experiential Learning. In, *Using Experience for Learning. Ch 3.*. Editors: Boud D. Cohen R. and Walker D. Milton Keynes. The Society for the Research into Higher Education. Open University Press.

Munhall P.L. and Oiler C. J. (1986) *Nursing Research. A Qualitative Perspective.* Connecticut. Appleton-Century -Crofts/Norwalk.

Ogier M.E. (1980) *A Study of the Leadership Style and Verbal Interactions of Ward Sisters with Learners.* London. Unpublished PhD Thesis. University of London.

Ogier M. E. (1982) *An Ideal Sister?* London. The Royal College of Nursing.

Orem D. (1980) *Nursing: Concepts of Practice.* (2nd Ed). New York. McGraw Hill.

Orton H.D. (1979) *Ward Learning Climate and Student Nurse Response.* Sheffield. CNAA Sheffield City Polytechnic. Unpublished MPhil thesis.

Orton H.D. (1981) *Learning Climate: A Study of the Role of the Ward Sister in Relation to Student Nurse Learning on the ward.* London. RCN.

Paton R. Chapman J. and Hamwee J (1985) People At Work. Unit 5. Block 11, Work Groups. *The Open University, T244. Managing in Organisations.* Milton Keynes, Open University Press.

Patton M. (1990) *Qualitative Evaluation and Research Methods.* (2nd Ed). London. Sage Publications.

Pearson A. and Vaughan B. (1986) *Nursing Models for Practice.* London. Heinemann Nursing.

Pembrey S. (1978) *The Role of the Ward Sister in the Management of Nursing.* Edinburgh. Unpublished PhD thesis University of Edinburgh.

Peplau H. (1952) *Interpersonal Relations in Nursing.* London, Macmillan Education Ltd.

Peplau H. (1988) *Interpersonal Relations in Nursing.* (2nd. Ed). London, Macmillan Education Ltd.

Peterson M.F. (1983) Co-workers and Hospital Staffs' work attitude: individual difference moderators. *Nursing Research. 32: 115-120*

Peterson, M. (1988) The norms and values held by three groups of nurses concerning psychosocial nursing practice. *International Journal of Nursing Studies.* 25. (2): 85-103.

Pfeiffer J. W. and Goodstein L.D. (1982) *The 1982 Annual for Facilitators, Trainers and Consultants.* San Diego. University Associates.

Pfeiffer J. W. and Jones J.E. (1974) *A Handbook of Structured Exercises for Human Relations Training.:* Vol. 1. La Jolla. University Associates.

Piaget J. (1971) *Psychology and Epistemology.* Harmonsworth. Penguin Books.

Pittenger O.E and Polanyi M (1971) *Learning Theory in Educational Practice.* New York, John Wiley & Sons. Gooding C.T.

Polanyi, M. (1966) *The Tacit Dimension.* Garden City, Doubleday. NY.

Polanyi, M. and Prosch H. (1975) *Meaning.* Chicago. The University of Chicago Press.

Pope M. & Denicolo P. (1986) Intuitive Theories-a Researcher's Dilemma: some practical methodological implications. *British Educational Research Journal.* 12, (2): 153-166.

Porritt L (1984) *Communication Choices for Nurses.* Melbourne. Churchill Livingstone.

Porter S. (1993) Nursing research conventions: Objectivity or Obfuscation? *Journal of Advanced Nursing.* (18): 137-143.

Pulsford D. (1993a) The reluctant participant in experiential Learning. *Nurse Education Today.* (13): 139-144.

Pulsford D. (1993b) The reluctant participant in experiential Learning. *Nurse Education Today.* (13): 145-148.

Rabkin J.G. and Struening E.L. (1976) Life Events, Stress and illness. *Science,* 194: 1013-1020.

Randell R. and Southgate J. (1980) *Co-operative and Community Group Dynamics: or Your Meetings Needn't be so Appalling.* London. Barefoot Books.

Reason P. and Rowan J. (1981) *Human Inquiry: A Sourcebook of New Paradigm Research.*(Eds) Chichester. John Wiley & Sons.

Reason P. (1987) On making sense-Chapter 10, In *Human Inquiry-A sourcebook of new paradigm research.* Reason P. & Rowan J. Eds. Chichester. John Wiley & Sons.

Reason P. and Marshell J (1987) Research as personal process. In Boud, D. Griffin, B.(Eds), *Appreciating Adult Learning: From the learner's perspective.* London: Kogan Page.

Reason P. (1988) *Co-operative Inquiry In Action: Developments in New Paradigm Research.* London. Sage Publication.

Reed J. and Procter S. (1993) *Nurse Education: A reflective approach.* (Eds) London. Edward Arnold and Hodder & Stoughton.

Reichardt C. and Cook T. (1979) Qualitative and Quantitative Methods in Evaluating Research. In Munhall, P.L. & Oiler, C.J. (Eds) (1986) *Nursing Research. A Qualitative Perspective.* Connecticut. Appleton-Century-Crofts/ Norwalk,

Reymolds B. (1985) Issues arising from Teaching Interpersonal Skills In Psychiatric Nurse Training. In Kagan C. M. (Ed). *Interpersonal Skills In Nursing. Research and Application.* Ch. 14. London. Croom Helm.

Roach S. (1984) *Caring: The Human Mode of Being. Implications for Nursing.* Perspectives in Caring, Monograph 1. Toronto. Faculty of Nursing, University of Toronto,

Roberts D. (1993) *Enpowerment Model.* Unpublished workshop demonstration. Metanioa. London.

RCN. (1987) *In Pursuit of Excellence.* published by a Working Party for the United Kingdom Central Council for Nurses and Midwives. London. RCN.

Rogers C.R. (1951) *Client-Centered Therapy.* London. Constable.

Rogers C.R. (1967) *On Becoming a Person.* London. Constable.

Rogers C.R. (1972)   The Facilitation of Significant Learning. In M.L. Silberman et al. (Eds) *The Psychology of Open Teaching and Learning.* Boston. Little Brown.

Rogers C.R. (1983) *Freedom to Learn for the 80's.* Columbus, Ohio. Merrill.

Roget P.M. (1962) *Roget's Thesaurus of English Words and Phrases.* Penguin Books. London. Harmondsworth.

Rolfe G. (1993)   Towards a theory of student-centred nurse education: overcoming the constraints of a professional curriculum. Nurse Education Today (1993) 13, 149-154

Roper N. Logan W. and Tierney A (1980)   *The Elements of Nursing.* Edinburgh: Churchill, Livingstone.

Rowan J. (1981) A dialectical paradigm for research. In Reason P. & Rowan J. Eds. *Human Inquiry: A Sourebook of New Paradigm Research.* Chapter 9. Chichester. John Wiley & Sons.

Rowan J. (1981) Issues of validity in new paradigm research. In Reason P. & Rowan J. Eds. *Human Inquiry: A Sourebook of New Paradigm Research.* Chapter 21. Chichester. John Wiley & Sons.

Rowan J. (1988) *Ordinary Ecstasy-Humanistic Psychology in Action* (2nd Ed) London/ New York. Routledge.

Roy C. (1976) *Introduction to Nursing: An Adaptation Model.* Old Tappen, New Jersey. Prentice Hall.

Salvage J. (1985) *The Politics of Nursing.* Oxford. Heinemann Nursing.

Sartre J.P. (1956) *Being and Nothingness.* New York: Philosophical Library.

Schein E. (1988) *Organisational Philosophy.* (3rd ed). London. Prentice Hall.

Schon D.A.(1983)   *The Reflective Practitioner: How Professionals Think in Action.* London. Temple Smith.

School of Nursing (1986)   *School of Nursing (S.O.N. (1) Curriculum Documents* (Internal document)

(1989) S.O.N. (2) (internal reports)

(1990) College of Nursing (1) (internal reports)

Schutz A. (1967)   *The Phenomenology of the Social World.* Evanston, IL. Northwestern University Press.

Schwartz P. and Ogilvy J. (1979) The Emergent Paradigm: Changing Patterns of Thought and Belief. In *Naturalistic Inquiry.* London. Sage Publications.

Seligman M. (1975) *Helplessness: on depression, development, and death.* San Francisco. W.H. Freeman and Company.

Sims D. (1981) From ethogeny to endogeny: how participants in research projects can end up doing research on their own awareness. In, Reason P. & Rowan J. (eds). *Human Inquiry, a sourcebook of new paradigm research.* Chapter 32. Chichester. John Wiley & Sons.

Sines D. (1993) Balance of Power (Mental Health) *Nursing Times.* 89, (46) pp.52-55

Skevington S (1984) *Understanding Nurses. The Social Psychology of Nursing.* (Ed). Chichester. John Wiley & Sons.

Skinner B.F. (1938) *The Behaviour of Organisms: An experimental Analysis.* New York. Appleton-Century-Crofts.

Smith P. (1988) The Emotional Labour of Nursing. *Nursing Times.* November 2, 84: 44.

Smith P. (1992) *The Emotional Labour of Nursing. How nurses care.* London. The Macmillan Press Ltd.

Spinelli E. (1989) *The Interpreted World-An Introduction to Phenomenological Psychology.* London. Sage Publications.

Stanford and Roark (1974*) Human Interaction in Education.* Boston. Allyn and Bacon.

Steinaker N. and Bell M. (1979) *The Experiential Taxonomy: A New Approach to Teaching and Learning.* New York. Academic Press.

Steiner C. (1990) *Scripts Peoples Live: Transactional analysis of life scripts.* 2nd Edition. New York, Grove Weidenfeld.

Stenhouse L. (1975) *An Introduction to Curriculum Research and Development.* London. Heinemann Education.

Stern P., Allen L. and Moxley P (1982) The Nurse as Grounded Theorist: History, process and uses. In, Munhall P. & Oiler C. (eds) *Nursing Research. A Qualitative Perspective.* Connecticut. Appleton-Century-Crofts/ Norwalk.

Stern P. (1985) Using Grounded Theory Method in Nursing Research. In Leininger M. (Ed) *Qualitative Research Methods in Nursing.* Ch. 10. W.B. Saunders Company Inc. USA.

Steven J.O. *(1971) Awareness: Exploring, Experimenting, Experiencing.* Moab, Utah: Real People Press.

Stewart I. and Joines V. (1987) *T A Today: A New Introduction to Transactional Analysis.* Nottingham and Chapel Hill.Lifespace Publishing.

Stockwell F. (1972) *The Unpopular Patient. RCN.* London.

Strauss A.L. (1987) *Qualitative Analysis for Social Scientists.* Cambridge University Press. Cambridge

Strauss A. and Corbin J. (1990) *Basics of Qualitative Research: Grounded theory procedures and techniques.* London. Sage Publications.

Sullivan H.S. (1948) *The Meaning of Anxiety in Psychiatry and in Life.* Washington DC. Williamson Alanson White Psychiatry Foundation.

Swanson J.M. (1986) Analyzing Data for Categories and Description. In Chenitz W. C. & Swanson J. M. (Eds) *From Practice to Grounded Theory: Qualitative Research in Nursing.* Ch. 10. Menlo Park. Addison-Wesley.

Tomlinson A. (1985) The Use of Experiential Methods in Teaching Interpersonal Skills to Nurses. In, Kagan C. (Ed) *Interpersonal Skills in Nursing. Research and Application.* Ch. 12. London. Croom Helm.

Tomlinson A. (1988) Communication for the Future-*Nursing 27* Aldwych Publishing-from the C.I.N.E. (Communication in Nurse Education project.) *Research by the University of Manchester and Kings College, University of London* (1982-85).

Torbert W.R. (1978) Educating toward Shared Purpose. The Theory and Practice of Liberating Structure. *Journal of Higher Education.* 49, (2): 109-135.

Tosey P. (1993) Module 1- Research. (unpublished) *Msc. in Change Agent Skills and Strategies.* Guildford. University of Surrey. Human Potential Resource Group.

Townsend I. (1983a) *Communication Skills-A Trainers Guide.* Sheffield. National Health Services. Learning Resources Unit.

Townsend I. (1983b) *Self-Awareness.* Sheffield. National Health Services. Learning Resources Unit.

Travelbee J. (1971) Interpersonal Aspects of Nursing. in *Understanding Nurses: The Social Psychology of Nursing.* Skevington Ed. ((1983)) John Wiley & Sons. Chichester.

Tuckman B.W (1965) Developmental sequences in small groups. *Psychological Bulletin,* 63, 384-399.

Turner B.A. (1981) Some Practical Aspects of Qualitative Data Analysis: One way of organising the cognitive processes associated with the generation of grounded theory. *Quality and Quantity Journal.* Vol 15(3) pp225-247.

Turner J.C. (1987) *Re-discovering the Social Group: A Self-categorisation Theory.* Oxford/New York. Basic Blackwell.

Turner J.H. (1988) *A Theory of Social Interaction.* Stanford. Polity Press.

Tyler R.W. (1949) *Basic Principles in Curriculum Instruction.* Chicago, University of Chicago Press.

UKCC (1983) *Nurse, Midwives and Health Visitors Rules.* London. Approved order (1983). Statutory instrument No.873.((1983)) Rule 18 (1). UKCC.

UKCC. (1984) *Code of Professional Conduct for the Nurse, Midwife and Health Visitor.* London. United Kingdom Central Council for Nursing, Midwifery and Health Visiting.

UKCC (1986) *Project 2000. A New Preparation For Practice.* London. United Kingdom Central Council (UKCC) for Nursing, Midwifery and Health Visiting.

United Nations General Assembly (1989) *The Conventions on the Rights of the Child (Children's rights).* Adopted by the United Nations General Assembly

Weil S and McGill I. (1989) *Making Sense of Experiential Learning: Diversity in Theory and Practice.* Milton Keynes. The Society for the Research into Higher Education & Open University Press.

West W.G. (1980) Access to Adolescent Deviants and Deviance". In Lofland J. & Lofland L. H. (1984). *Analysing Social Settings: A Guide to Qualitative*

Observation and Analysis. (2nd.ed). Belmont. Wadsworth Publishing Company.

Wilde V. (1992)   Controversial Hypotheses on the relationship between researcher and informant in qualitative research. *Journal of Advanced Nursing.* 17: 234-242.

Williamson B. (1979) Education, Social Structure and Development. London. Macmillan Press.

Wilmot S. (1993) Ethics, agency and empowerment in nurse education. *Nurse Education Today.* 13, 189-195.

Wilson-Barnett J. (1978)   Patients' emotional responses to barium x-rays. *Journal of Advanced Nursing.* 3, 37-46.

Worchel S. (1992)   *Group Process and Productivity.* (Eds) London. Sage Publication

Yalom I. (1985)   *The Theory and Practice of Group Psychotherapy.* 3rd ed. Basic Books. USA.